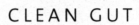

CLEAN GUT

**Also by Alejandro Junger**

*Clean*

# CLEAN GUT

The Breakthrough Plan for
Eliminating the Root Cause of Disease
and Revolutionizing Your Health

Alejandro Junger

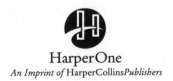

HarperOne
*An Imprint of* HarperCollins*Publishers*

HarperOne

This book contains advice and information relating to health care. It should be used to supplement rather than replace the advice of your doctor or another trained health professional. If you know or suspect that you have a health problem, it is recommended that you seek your physician's advice before embarking on any medical program or treatment. Before doing the Clean Gut program, check with your doctor to make sure it is a good fit for you. Do not do the Clean Gut program if you are: under the age of 18, are pregnant or nursing, or have an allergy to any supplement mentioned in this book. All efforts have been made to assure the accuracy of the information contained in this book as of the date of publication. The publisher and the author disclaim liability for any medical outcomes that may occur as a result of applying the methods suggested in this book.

FIRST EDITION

*Interior Design by Laura Lind Design*
*Illustrations by Robert Pereida*

Library of Congress Cataloging-in-Publication Data.

Junger, Alejandro.
Clean Gut: the breakthrough plan for eliminating the root cause of disease and revolutionizing your health / Alejandro Junger.
pages cm
ISBN 978–0–06–207586–4
1. Gastrointestinal system—Diseases—Popular works. 2. Digestive organs—Diseases—Popular works. 3. Chronic diseases—Prevention—Popular works.
I. Title.
RC801.J86 2013
616.3—dc23 2013000286

14 15 16 17 RRD(H) 10 9 8 7 6 5

*I dedicate this book to Carla, my wife, my soulmate.*
*Cuka, my heart is in your hands.*
*It could not be in better hands . . . I love you.*

# Contents

# CHAPTER ONE

# The Root Cause
# of Disease

My first lesson in good medicine came when I was a young boy growing up in Uruguay, many years before I started medical school. It arrived from the unlikeliest of people. I used to follow around a gardener named Fermin as he tended to the plants in our home. I noticed that when he saw an unhealthy tree, he spent most of his time inspecting the roots and the soil around them. He only took a quick glance at the leaves. He would then devise a plan: more water, less water, fertilizer, pest removal, or some other remedy he kept in his gardening toolbox. I always wondered why he wasted his time down there around the roots when the problem was clearly up here on the leaves. I mean, I was actually staring at the problem!

When I asked Fermin why he cared so much about the roots, he simply smiled. "Boy," he said, "that's the way nature designed it. Your tree's health and disease start in its roots." My first thought at the time, if I remember correctly, was *yeah, whatever,* but I couldn't argue with Fermin's results. Time and time again Fermin took care of most problems by changing the conditions around the roots. The leaves always returned lush and green. Fermin was a good gardener, and a wise man.

The reason I say this was my first lesson in good medicine is because after eight years of medical school, six years of training, and another fifteen years of practice, I came to the conclusion that good medicine is very much like good gardening. Imagine you have a tree you love. One day you notice its leaves have turned brown. They will, you understand, soon wither and fall off. Imagine now that you call an expert who, after close examination of the leaves, recommends that you paint them green and attach them back to their branches so the tree can at least appear to be healthy. Everyone would agree that's crazy. If you want to get your tree truly healthy, you can't just cover up the problem. You need to get to the root of it. And just like Fermin used to say, the problem is most likely in the roots.

While I was in medical school the trend in modern medicine was to specialize and super specialize. Doctors became experts in one organ or even one part of one organ. More advanced technology helped not only detect problem areas, but also treat them. The advances of science were mesmerizing, and people held the practice of medicine in high regard. The great irony of our success, however, was that we only got better at painting the leaves. We went way beyond gardeners who paint the brown leaves green. We cut out whole branches and replaced them with healthier ones. Or built artificial branches and leaves altogether. We got so good at attacking individual diseases and symptoms we forgot to look at their root causes.

Take the medical community's response to inflammation, for instance. After I completed my training as a cardiologist, in 1998, scientists started to notice that all chronic diseases—

regardless of how different each disease seemed or where each disease presented in the body—shared one common condition: inflammation. Identified as a precursor of disease, the medical establishment turned its attention to fighting it. Inflammation quickly became the "new disease on the block." Hundreds of articles, studies, and books were written about it, and entire industries were born in the fight against it. While the fight against inflammation helped many people alleviate their suffering, it is really just the first symptom of disease. The fight against it is really just another example of modern medicine's attempt to keep individual leaves vibrant and green while the plant is dying. We still need to get to the root of disease.

*Clean Gut* does this. Before chronic disease, there is inflammation; but before inflammation comes gut dysfunction. Anti-inflammation treatments help, but gut repair corrects the problem right at its source.

In these pages I reveal how your overall health is connected to a singular area of the body, your gut. I explain how the root of almost all chronic diseases also starts in your gut. You will discover that most of the "diseases" being diagnosed in epidemic proportions—such as heart disease, cancer, autoimmune diseases, insomnia, depression, asthma, diabetes, and arthritis—can all be traced back to your injured and irritated gut.

Even if you have not been diagnosed with a specific disease, many of the minor ailments you may be suffering from—such as tiredness, aches and pains, allergies, mood swings, lack of libido, bad breath, body odor, eczema, and constipation—may also be directly related to gut dysfunction. In addition, a damaged gut will lead to premature aging. These symptoms are often justified and attributed to the unavoidable wear and tear of your aging body, but they are ultimately directly related to the health of your gut and can be reversed by a gut repair program.

In fact, most health issues affecting the world's populace today are the result of a disrupted, damaged gut. It is critical that we make this vitally important information and health tool available to everyone. *Clean Gut* is a proven path to avoiding disease and reclaiming your own power to get truly healthy.

In my first book, *Clean,* I explained how the toxic chemicals we are exposed to, and the toxic conditions we create in our lives, are responsible for many of our health problems. Nobody escapes this reality. This is true now more than ever. There are great possible benefits for most people when they learn how to activate and support their bodies' detoxifying organs and systems. The twenty-one-day Clean cleanse has helped thousands do just that.

In *Clean Gut,* I share a powerful new program, a critical tool in preemptively attacking and eliminating disease at the root. We do not have to wait until we are sick to get healthy. Let me explain. The most common toxins come in our food, and your gut bears the brunt of these toxins. Even toxins that are absorbed through your skin and lungs will eventually end up causing havoc in your gut. Take a shower with unfiltered water in any city in America and you will end up with some amount of chlorine circulating in your blood, which will reach the cells at the lining of your gut and negatively affect the gut's good bacteria. The reality is that life these days is *not* gut friendly.

It is unquestionable that the state of human health is in crisis. We are sick and getting sicker. Everyone seems to be suffering from something, getting tests done, taking over-the-counter and prescription medications. Chronic diseases are on the rise. Too many people are diagnosed with a growing number of diseases. It is out of control. When I was in medical school, I saw many patients with cancer, but this was not the case in my personal life. Today, however, many of my friends have cancer and many more people I know are being diagnosed with it. Diseases that were rare in the 1980s, such as autoimmune diseases, are now global epidemics.

Not only is the state of human health in crisis, the state of our medical system is also about to collapse. Doctors have no reservations about spitting out a diagnosis, ordering sophisticated tests, and prescribing treatments, which include drastic surgeries and radical combinations of prescription drugs to silence our symptoms. These combinations of chemicals are often effective in suppressing symptoms but are frequently all too toxic. Many health issues, and in some cases death, are caused by treatments given to patients by the most competent doctors.

A pill for an ill to suppress symptoms is a lot like painting the brown leaves green for a sick tree. It is just bad gardening. And it doesn't work. I talk to people all over the world, and there is a general frustration with the current state of medicine. People are disappointed by their doctors and upset by the lack of information and real, lasting solutions. We were taught to trust physicians and to be fascinated by and grateful to science, but this kind of blind faith in the medical profession is beginning to wane.

There are still many of us who believe we are diagnosing more diseases because we are constantly getting better at it through better science and technology. It is far too easy to accept the current state of medical care and assume that without it things would probably be much worse. We are told and expected to believe that diseases are a combination of bad luck and bad genes—mainly that diseases happen when the body is doing something wrong.

Symptoms are grouped into syndromes, which are classified by systems. A series of laboratory tests are often necessary to confirm a diagnosis. Treatment is usually a standardized plan, which mostly consists of surgeries and medications. It doesn't matter which patient has a particular disease but what particular disease a patient has. Modern medicine offers the same treatment for the same diagnosis no matter who you are.

It doesn't have to be this way. By focusing on gut health, you can eliminate disease at the root, and protect your health for the long term. Even if you have followed Clean or another program that focuses on detoxification and have already eliminated the majority of your exposure to toxic chemicals, your gut may still be in need of further repair. Organic, chemical-free food can also negatively affect your gut's health if eaten in the wrong combinations, frequency, or quantity. Certain foods—such as sugar, caffeine, and dairy—that you may have not yet identified could be toxic triggers, which initiate a cascade of reactions that erode your health from the roots up.

All these negative and toxic influences disrupt the gut. Simply reverting to a "healthy" diet is not enough. Special measures must be taken and specific conditions must be met in order to aid our bodies in their attempts to repair themselves. This is what we do with other organs in our bodies when the damage is beyond "natural self-repair."

Within the medical community, the word "gut" is a loosely defined term. It's more often used as just another way to talk about our intestines. When I use the word gut, however, I refer to a lot more than just the body's digestive tube. I mean the living organisms inside the gut, the intestinal flora, and the immune and nervous systems within and around the walls of the intestines. The body doesn't make a distinction between these different parts. Nor should we. Together, these different organs and tissues make up the gut, one of the most complex and important instruments in your body. Your health and well-being depend on all these parts working in concert, at their highest levels, in more ways than you can imagine. It's simple, really: if you learn about how your gut works and understand how to repair and keep it clean, you will achieve vibrant, long-lasting health.

The gut performs essential functions in the body. The different organs of the gut, while working interdependently, remain in constant communication with each other through nerves and hormones. How the gut functions has both a direct and indirect effect on every single cell in the human body, from the cells in your bone marrow deep inside your bones to the hair and skin on the surface. Often dysfunctions in the gut cause symptoms in the unlikeliest parts of the body. A rash on the skin, for instance. When you notice a rash, you consult a dermatologist. Because the rash is something you can see and feel, chances are the dermatologist will focus his or her attention there and prescribe a cream to eliminate the rash or the accompanying itchiness. In other words, the dermatologist is simply painting the brown leaves green. This is just one example of how a dysfunction in the gut presents itself as a different symptom somewhere—anywhere—else in the body. There are countless others. As I regularly tell patients, the gut is the body's great trickster, hiding in plain sight. It fools almost everyone, including doctors and even gastroenterologists, into thinking that it's perfectly fine. That the *real* problem is somewhere else.

The medical establishment continues to minimize or entirely overlook gut health in the way I talk about it here. The state of the art of prevention in gastroenterology is a colonoscopy for early polyp detection and excision. Doctors are constantly searching for a link between specific organs and certain types of illness, disease, and germs without thinking how the gut factors in. Or they focus on the organs that seem to have more of an immediate impact on our immediate survival, such as the heart, which has to continue beating, the kidneys, which have to filter the blood, or the brain, which has to fire neurons. Modern medicine continues as "a pill for an ill" industry largely because very few doctors pay close attention to the gut. Just as the secret to a lush garden starts in the plants' roots, the body's health begins in the gut, its own internal roots. The gut is the center of health, illness, and dysfunction. If you want to figure out why your leaves are turning brown, so to speak, look at your gut.

*Clean Gut* will help your body repair your gut. No matter your current state of health, you will benefit from this program. Based on the four Rs of functional medicine—Remove, Replace, Reinoculate, and Repair—the Clean Gut program is divided into two distinct phases. The first phase is a twenty-one-day diet, which focuses on eating easily digestible and low-sugar foods while removing the kinds of food that lead to gut dysfunction. It also includes necessary supplements that will address the different aspects of gut repair that your body needs outside help with. The second—and crucial—phase is a seven-day reintroduction process, the purpose of which is to identify the foods that do you the most harm. These toxic triggers, as I call them, must be identified to fully restore and maintain gut health. Combined, this is a comprehensive program that can be easily integrated into your daily life and has the potential to heal and restore the area in your body that is most taxed by your everyday life: your gut.

We are all walking around with damaged guts and, to different degrees, suffering the consequences in our day-to-day and long-term health. Without an optimally functioning gut, we simply don't have a chance of achieving true long-lasting health. When we repair the gut and eliminate the root of disease, however, major and minor symptoms disappear, and we discover what it means to be truly healthy.

For some, it may be a very subtle improvement, but subtle improvement can be phenomenal. A good friend of mine lives a really healthy life. Jimmy eats well and exercises regularly. He says he always feels great. But, as my friend, he's had to listen to me describe what I observe in so many people. Eventually, he got curious and decided to try the Clean Gut program. After the program, he described that he was breathing more deeply and slowly, and the air in his lungs felt fresh and new, unlike anything he had ever experienced before. He described being more alert and aware and feeling that breathing gave him more satisfaction and pleasure. The result was a better and clearer experience of every minute of the day.

For others, the results will be more far-reaching, such as it was for Magdalena. She had always felt tired and had many debilitating symptoms: dry mouth, dry eyes, joint pain, multiple infections lasting weeks, and many others. She visited many doctors until one finally diagnosed Behçet's syndrome, an autoimmune disease. She was told that the treatment for the severity of her disease was methotrexate, a chemotherapy agent also used for many types of cancer. What frightened Magdalena the most was that this treatment greatly reduced her chances of getting pregnant. She contacted me from Uruguay shortly thereafter. I put her on the Clean Gut program as a trial before she started her methotrexate treatment. After twenty-one days, the majority of Magdalena's symptoms had completely disappeared or were significantly reduced. Magdalena reported that she had never felt so strong, so good, or so healthy in her life. She decided against the treatment and is instead focusing on getting pregnant.

Whether we are just repairing inevitable minor damage or eliminating diseases at their root, improving gut health has rewarded my patients with a new level of health and vibrancy they never imagined. This approach to gut repair is the most powerful healing tool in my medical toolbox, and it has helped many of my patients all over the world. Now you can do it by following the Clean Gut program as outlined in chapter 6. Restore your gut's health and stop disease from the get-go—or, more accurately, from the gut-go!

Just as *Clean* was not a product of multimillion-dollar clinical trials or a pharmaceutical company sponsorship, *Clean Gut* is also the result of my personal, spiritual, and professional journey, a journey that led me around the world, all the way back to my first lesson with Fermin.

# CHAPTER TWO

# The Patient, the Teacher, and the Doctor

I didn't just wake up one day and decide to reinvent myself as a doctor. I was desperately looking for solutions for my own health problems.

After an intense residency at Beekman, New York University's Downtown Hospital, and a grueling cardiology fellowship at Lenox Hill Hospital, where I ran the cardiac intensive care unit during my nights on call, my health was in ruins. Six straight years of endless workdays, sleepless nights, and a steady diet of microwavable dinners and fast food had done a number on my system. I was exhausted and overweight. I was depressed and in constant discomfort. My seasonal allergies, which developed shortly after I arrived in New York, had turned into a year-round torture of sneezing, itching, sniffling, and coughing. What had started as mild constipation—the result of takeout meals, vending-machine snacks, nurses' potlucks, and food from the hospital cafeteria—had worsened

into abdominal pain, cramps, bloating, and explosive episodes
of diarrhea, which sometimes occurred a few minutes after a
meal. My lips blistered whenever I spent more than a few hours
in the sun. I had hemorrhoids. On most days, I couldn't function. To be honest, I didn't *want* to function.

I felt like giving up. So I decided to seek help from my peers.
I visited three specialists: an allergist, a gastroenterologist, and
a psychiatrist. I ended up with seven prescription medications
for three different diagnoses: severe allergies, irritable bowel
syndrome (IBS), and depression. The idea of taking chemicals
for the rest of my life to silence my symptoms in order to function didn't make sense. So, I started to look for answers outside my world of hospitals and medical offices. This journey led
to the first of my three aha moments, three clarifying visions
about life—and health—that even today continue to inform
my holistic approach to medicine and health.

## The Journey Begins:
## A Sneak Preview into Awakening

Since my most disturbing symptom was depression, I made
appointments with therapists, counselors, and social workers. I
also read self-help books by Nathaniel Branden, Gay Hendricks,
and Wayne Dyer, as well as Shakti Gawain's work on creative
visualization. My search eventually led me to a school of meditation, where I learned that one can achieve a state of uninterrupted presence through meditation, a state that emotionally
feels like uninterrupted peace. While there, I got a taste of this
state during an intensive weekend meditation course with the
school's teacher, a radiant Indian woman who teaches these
principles by example.

The weekend intensive alternated between chanting sessions, silent mediation sessions, and sessions during which other students and the school's monks shared their personal experiences. I attended all the sessions and did my best to meditate during the periods of silent meditation. But nothing was happening. I couldn't even sit still for a few minutes with my eyes closed. At one point, a student from France started speaking about how meditation had transformed his life. His story was very similar to my own. He'd been a happy kid but then his mind got dark and full of negative, racing thoughts. As I identified with everything this man was saying, something really strange took place. Suddenly, the whole hall grew dark, closing in on me as if I were getting tunnel vision. I could see only the French man's face, which then began to move closer and closer to me. He was looking straight at me and coming closer in my tunnel until *bam!* I switched physical places with him. He was me, and I was him. But I wasn't really him. I was just experiencing his vantage point, looking out from his eyes and seeing my own body in the distance. When he finished talking, and all the people in the room started clapping, I was immediately back in my own body looking at the French man acknowledging the applause from the crowd. I thought I might have had a hallucination.

Sweating profusely, I quickly got up and went to the cafeteria to sit down, drink something, and pull myself together. Prema, a longtime resident of the school, approached me and said I looked pale. She asked if I was okay. After I told her what had happened, she urged me to return to the next chanting session. On our way back, in an empty corridor, we came face to face with the meditation teacher. The three of us stopped, and the teacher looked me in the eyes and asked me my name and what I did for a living. I told her I was a cardiologist. "Oh, the heart," she said knowingly with a big smile on her face. And without another word, she smacked me on the chest and walked away. I lost sensation in my legs first, and then my whole body. Past, present, and future all merged into one overwhelming sense of quiet, joy, and timelessness.

This was the moment of my spiritual rebirth. When my meditation teacher hit my heart, I went into a state that is very hard to describe. My consciousness was everywhere, and I felt an overwhelming sensation of peace, one I had never known before. This feeling lasted for what seemed an eternity but was, in reality, probably just under a minute. I felt a pull on my hand and slowly noticed that Prema was shaking me and asking me if I was okay. She wiped the tears (of joy) from my face and led me back to the hall.

Over the next two weeks, I spontaneously experienced many similar episodes. Longing to understand what I was experiencing, I drove back to the school many times and talked to people, watched videos, and read the school's books. Based on what I learned, I was experiencing a sneak preview of what my inner divinity would be like. When we receive initiation, we gain entry to our inner spiritual realms as the coiled-up kundalini energy at the base of our spines begins uncoiling and pushing upward through some seventy-two thousand energy channels called the nadis, which connect the chakras from bottom to top. Then, through practice, our own spiritual awareness unfolds. The energy eventually reaches our crown chakra, the sahasrara, the gate to higher consciousness, where we can experience clarity and have perception beyond ordinary sight.

About a month after my first taste of a calm, fully present mind, the meditation school announced that it needed a doctor at its mother school in India. Its first-aid station needed a new physician, as many of the monks were getting sick and the previous doctor had left. I filled out the application and sent it in. A few days later, I was asked, "When can you come?"

•  •  •

India opened up a whole new world for me, literally and figuratively. In India, I studied much more than meditation. I was introduced to new healing modalities and learned more about yoga, meditation, Indian philosophies, and spirituality. I also ran a clinic with practitioners from many modalities. My job involved directing a team of volunteer health practitioners from around the world, who treated the large population at this particular meditation school. We used a converted school bus as our traveling hospital to the surrounding villages—some of the poorest places on the planet, where we encountered scores of patients in need of our assistance. The experience was one of the most rewarding in my life. I would have never discovered it had I stayed on the traditional path for a doctor like me in America.

For the first time ever I was practicing integrative medicine, a term that I hadn't known before, and it felt much more like the vision I had of being a doctor when I was much younger. It was truly integrative by every definition of that word, as my team wasn't just filled with classically trained physicians like me. There were ayurvedic and Chinese medicine doctors, nurses, chiropractors, massage therapists, acupuncturists, hands-on healers, and meditation instructors, among others. They all contributed a slightly different approach and philosophy. I was amazed by what I witnessed. I heard other doctors explain their perspectives on illness and health in ways that made total sense, even though my formal education had never taught me these perspectives. I watched patients heal by using herbs, eating or avoiding certain foods, and receiving massage.

Of course there were cases that relied on Western medicine's use of drugs and surgery, but no sooner had I immersed myself in this environment of integrative healing than I began to realize that there wasn't any such thing as "alternative" or even "traditional." It was, simply put, common sense. In every case, we looked for and addressed the root cause of imbalances in the body. Unlike the focus of Western medicine, we did more than just treat symptoms and try to hold them at bay. We cared for the body as a whole, removed its obstacles, and provided whatever it lacked in order to shift it back into a gear that would support and maintain health. More often than not, I saw that people could restore their bodies back to health without drugs. One of the most powerful tools we had was food. It was the first time I began to understand the old proverb that food is medicine. Looking back now, I see that my time in India prepared me to realize the far-reaching effects of gut health on total health.

My year in India was transformative, to say the least. No longer did I perceive lines or boundaries between "Eastern" and "Western" medicine. No longer did I view medicine as divided into different categories or schools of thought, such as "complementary" and "conventional." To me, all the medical traditions and practices were one, which I called "open-minded medicine." The goal of a doctor like me was to bring the best from every tradition and, without judgment, use this vast body of knowledge to serve every person as a unique individual. In addition to my shift of perspective on doctoring, I physically changed. Many of the physical ailments that had plagued me in America had improved.

When I returned to the United States, I wanted to share my experience and new knowledge with my Western colleagues, but I didn't know how to do that or where to begin. I traveled to the meditation school for a brief residency. My confusion over what to do next was compounded by the fact that the school of meditation was planning to build a new hospital in India, so I was tempted to return and help direct the whole project. But I wasn't even sure that I wanted to continue practicing medicine. I had lost my north. It was 1999, and I was thirty-five years old. A friend recommended that I speak to the meditation teacher, so I requested a private meeting. Before I was granted the meeting I was asked to talk to one of the school's monks, who said, "It's great to talk to the master, but are you ready to take her command?" So I went back to my room to think and meditate. Remembering the chest-smacking state she had put me in before, I was left with no doubt of her authenticity and I felt ready to take on anything, no matter the consequences.

One never visits such a master empty handed, so I bought her some flowers and a coconut, which I offered as I bowed and kneeled before her. After she thanked me for my work in India, I explained my confusion. "I came to America to study and train to be a great cardiologist, but now I am lost. Should I stay in the school? Should I continue to practice medicine?"

She simply replied that I had to do what I had to do. I had to go out in the world and do my work, and my work was doing whatever I do with an open heart. She went on to say that perhaps I'd find something that would help a lot of people. Something I hadn't studied in medical school, but because I'm a doctor people wouldn't think it was hokey-pokey. And that maybe what I'd find would become known around the world. Little did I know then that what she was referring to was my Clean community, which would begin to take shape ten years after this encounter.

At the end of our conversation, my teacher said, "Now, go." But as I stood up to leave, she told me to wait a minute, looked me intensely in the eyes, and calmly said that she had two commands for me: Don't worry. Don't hurry. Then she gestured with her hand and said I could go. Just as I made my way toward the door in the back, I suddenly felt her hand on my shoulder, as if she'd magically teleported herself from the front of the room. She turned me around, it seemed, and added forcefully, "Alejandro! I mean it. Don't worry, and don't hurry."

I left the meditation school and returned to Manhattan. Oddly enough, things seemed to fall into place, even though I never made formal plans. In a day or so, I traveled to Los Angeles to be the best man at a friend's wedding. After the celebrations, I stayed at the newlyweds' house, dogsitting for them while they went on their honeymoon. As I started to get to know the neighborhood, I put together a résumé to send all over. I had a special visa to work in underserved areas, and I responded to the needs of a practice in the city of Joshua Tree, a couple hours east of Los Angeles, near Palm Springs. So I moved to the desert of California and joined the practice. It was a busy and lucrative practice, but I quickly realized I was back in the rat race I had tried so hard to escape. On average, I spent only about seven minutes with each patient, usually prescribing medications, while ordering test after test and procedure after procedure. It was virtually impossible to maintain a peaceful well-being amid all the commitments and responsibilities. They swallowed me whole in my new position as an attending cardiologist in a busy practice with admitting privileges in the four local hospitals, each of which had its own pile of bureaucracy to contend with. In addition to the effects of punishing commutes in the car, responding to beepers morning, noon, and night, and tending to emergencies, I juggled the weight of keeping the practice profitable while simultaneously making rounds of wards and intensive care units. I felt like I was always moving at warp speed and had no time to catch up with myself, let alone spend any meaningful time with my patients.

This experience was so counter to how I'd learned to care for patients in India. I was now participating in a system designed to encourage more tests, drugs, and surgery rather than take a step back and try to understand the root cause of disease before addressing physical symptoms. I also felt entrapped by a grueling medical system that was more about money and politics than true health *care*. I wanted to change this ingrained, "sick" system, which supported sickness rather than wellness, but I met too many obstacles.

## My Second Aha Moment: Global Toxicity

Before long, the health I had regained in India took another turn for the worse. As the stress, late-night dinners, and cafeteria food once again assaulted me, so too did my irritable bowel syndrome and depression. I often wondered if I was any better off than many of my patients. This time, however, it wasn't a visit to a foreign country that rescued me. It was a surprise visit by my friend Eric, who arrived ten days after he'd completed a detox program at a holistic center located just a few minutes from my home in Palm Springs. The moment I opened the door to see his shining, joyful face was one I'll always remember. Just ten days earlier, he'd been his usual bloated, overweight, sallow-skinned self—an overworked movie producer who, like me, had a body that had taken a beating from a life filled with too many competing demands and a dead diet. Eric was eager to tell me about his experience. He'd abandoned his usual routine of restaurant meals, coffee, and all-night movie shoots for a retreat based on green juices, colonics, massage, sunshine, yoga, and meditation. I was shocked by the changes in him and needed to find out what he had done in this place. I wanted to understand what had happened to him.

I immediately went to the center, called We Care Spa, and met its visionary founder and owner, Susana Belen. I was astounded by this woman's insights and knowledge about health, without her being a doctor. I worked out a way to embark on a two-week program while continuing to fulfill my medical duties. I drove there on my lunch breaks to pick up supplements and jars of fresh juices. I received colonic hydrotherapy treatments daily to help flush out all the toxins that were being released from my tissues via my intestines. By the third day of the detox program, my energy was returning and my constant hunger and headaches were dissipating. By the seventh day, my IBS had vanished. At the end of the cleansing protocol, my depression had lifted and I'd shed fifteen pounds. I felt amazing, just like my friend. And people noticed. Colleagues wanted to know how I looked ten years younger, as if I'd found the fountain of youth. Perhaps I had.

As I learned while in India, the body's different parts, systems, and functions are all interconnected, which helps explain how bringing balance back to my body as a whole through detox managed to remedy so many of my problems. It took this experience, however, to remind me of the importance of honoring the body as a unit and weeding out toxic insults to any single part of it, which throw it all out of whack. From my mood and general energy level to my medical conditions and chronic symptoms, I witnessed a renewal of health through diet alone, as if my body had physically and emotionally reset itself without drugs. And all it took to restore my health was a simple, straightforward protocol that allowed my body to naturally cleanse and detoxify my cells.

This was my second aha moment. I had had another awakening, a radical shift in thought about how to care for my body. I became aware of the toxicity of our planet and the consequences to our health. Modern medicine had taught me that my set of symptoms—mood, energy, allergies, IBS—were all separate problems for which different solutions were necessary. But the detox program helped me understand that the body can repair itself from the inside out with just food and water.

Word traveled quickly through my circle of friends and family about my change, and I started inviting people to stay with me in Palm Springs and embark on a similar program using the juice blends I was making at home. I kept experimenting with all kinds of juices while going to We Care Spa on the weekends to study and speak with other people. My home got busy; at one point there was a waiting list for people to come stay with me. It was like I was living a double life: during the day I was a cardiologist and on weekends I was engrossed in learning more at We Care and immersing myself in all I could about detoxification. Eventually, I began lecturing at the spa to share what I was finding. Indeed, I was in the open about being a cardiologist during my working hours, but in my free time I secretly studied cleansing and detox at the We Care Spa. I felt like I was in the holistic "closet."

## Finding My Home as a Doctor

While all this learning and discovering was going on, however, things were getting bad at work. Suffice it to say, the politics of the practice where I worked worsened to the point that I decided to quit two months before making partner. It was a blessing in disguise, for I immediately became more involved with We Care as a medical consultant and lecturer. This also allowed me to move to Los Angeles, where I could expand my knowledge and reach in the community, as well as surround myself with a bigger city filled with progressive thinkers and leaders in health movements. During the week, I worked at a clinic in West Los Angeles with a Chinese medical practitioner and a chiropractor. Each weekend, I drove to We Care to continue studying and lecturing.

At this time, I discovered functional medicine, when a colleague urged me to attend its introductory course, Applying Functional Medicine in Clinical Practice (AFMCP). This became yet another turning point for me. The rapidly growing field of functional medicine translates the Eastern paradigm of health to fit the Western terminology and tools with incredibly effective results. It was the missing link for me. Before being introduced to functional medicine what I'd been seeing at We Care seemed like magic, because I hadn't learned about these methods of cleansing and detoxification during my years in medical school or my post-graduate training. But now I was finding out why it was an important key to health, and especially how building health through dietary change was possible. I was finally making the connections between the ancient traditions and the new scientific studies that could explain the biochemistry of detoxification in rich detail. The proof from science was there. The transformations I was witnessing weren't magical. They were real, and the Institute for Functional Medicine had already done the scientific research to demonstrate what I was seeing from a medical, clinical standpoint, using the same language I'd learned in medical school.

This was my third aha moment. I said to myself, *I've found my home as a scientist; I am a functional medicine doctor.* My practice as a doctor slowly shifted as I began to treat patients using a much wider perspective, armed with a toolkit that went beyond the traditional methods prescribed by my American medical colleagues. Although I had returned from India with the intention of blending the knowledge I'd gained there with Western medicine, it wasn't really possible for me to do that previously. But the stakes were finally high enough for me to follow through on my promise.

I continued to go to We Care on weekends and give lectures. People also signed up for private consultations. I guided many different people through their juice-fasting experiences, and helped individuals create a long-term health plan they could sustain. I sent many individuals from Los Angeles to We Care too, where they had similar transformations through their detoxification program and came back with a new lease on life.

But constantly commuting to Palm Springs on a weekly basis ran its course. At the same time, I was having difficulties achieving the same results with the people who wanted to stay in Los Angeles on the program compared to the guests of We Care. Juicing worked well in a spa setting, where life was on hold. But that wasn't the case in the city. So, I started to research and design a way to make the program work any-where, including a busy city like Los Angeles, where people are constantly bombarded by toxic elements. It's one thing to check into a luxurious spa, where everything is relatively con-trolled for you, it's another to try to live a clean life at home and work in the reality of modern society.

My experience at We Care inspired me to develop the Clean program, which has helped hundreds of thousands of people restore their bodies' natural ability to heal itself. As you can imagine, I was at the top of my game and felt amazing. I had started a movement that could change the health of the world. Every day I ran on the beach, meditated, and enjoyed my community of like-minded people, who kept me super fit.

Everything was working unbelievably well. I was in the best shape of my life. But then a series of events happened that radically changed the course of my life—yet again and forever. In fact, what transpired is proof that you can have all the answers for physical health, but then life unexpectedly throws you a curve ball.

I met a woman with whom I started a relationship. Within a few months, we decided to have a baby. My daughter, Grace, was born on May 25, 2006. Three months after that, my romantic relationship with Grace's mother ended and I moved out. I was crushed. The pain of the separation from my daughter nearly killed me. Within weeks, I went from feeling superhuman to being near death in my bedroom with double pneumonia. The Chinese believe the lungs are the seat of grief, and this was my validation. Before I could address my deep depression, however, I had to take care of my worsening lung infection. But even that was hard for me to do because, believe it or not, I had no medical insurance. So I tried to sweat it out at home. It wasn't until my dear friend Richard came over and lifted me off my bed to take me to his home that I found my next lifeline. Richard put me on a regimen of antibiotics and chicken soup, as well as listened to me for hours as I poured my heart out. I slowly began to recover. I had to learn the lesson again: not all doctors are healers, and not all healers are doctors. My time in India had taught me this fundamental lesson, but somehow I'd forgotten it until this near-death experience.

When I'd fully recovered, I was lured back to New York. Richard plainly said to me that I needed a new environment where I couldn't wallow in my misery of the separation from my daughter. It didn't take long for me to make connections in New York, with my friend's help, and soon enough I was invited to work in a prestigious medical practice. I tried to get back to the routine I'd had in California, because I wanted to feel fit and superhuman again. But it was hard—much harder than I had anticipated. Ironically, it was during this time that I wrote *Clean,* yet I myself couldn't execute all the tenets I was teaching. My environment in New York antagonized every effort to live up to my personal philosophy. I fell back into old patterns of eating poorly and overworking myself, I stopped exercising, and I lacked the community that was so essential to living healthily in California. I spent countless hours in airplanes and hotels as I returned to Los Angeles to spend as much time with my daughter as possible. I didn't have the support system that I needed to truly restore and sustain my health.

It almost always takes a crisis for people to make big changes in their lives for the better of their health, and I am no exception. I call it the "eviction notice"—the diagnosis that suddenly gives us the motivation to change. There are those who try to force change every January with the ringing in of a new year. There are those who get motivated thanks to an upcoming event, such as a wedding, or the desire to start a family. For me, I needed to find my own extraordinary motivation, which would push me down a path to wellness again. I didn't necessarily have a serious eviction notice, and I wasn't planning to attend a reunion anytime soon. But I was on the lookout for a life partner, a woman with whom I could share my life. And that's what it took to yank me out of my health-depleting rut in New York.

It all started with a phone consultation from Australia, with a man who would become a dear friend of mine and who set me up with Carla, who is now my wife and the mother of my two other children. This man had heard about the amazing results patients were experiencing doing my program and he wanted me to personally guide him, which I did. We became fast friends. When his wife showed me a photograph of her best friend, I instantly fell deeply in love with the woman in the picture. And I immediately resolved to clean up my health before meeting my future wife. So I started the Clean program, and by the time I flew to Argentina, where my friends have a farm and were hosting Carla as a guest, I was back in tip-top shape, physically, mentally, and emotionally. Five months after our first semi-blind date, Carla and I married in Australia and then moved to Los Angeles so we could be close to Grace. *Clean* was becoming a huge success and I was busy building my Clean community throughout the United States.

## My Journey Continues: Getting Back to the Roots

Despite the program's success, however, I realized that detoxification alone was not fully repairing my patients' health. I came to the conclusion that even after a successful cleansing and detox program, a person's gut can often remain damaged, still in need of repair. This compelled me to focus my attention on gut repair and learn as much as I could about it. Because the body's systems, organs, tissues, and cells are interconnected, it's impossible to go through a good detox program without fixing gut damage at some level, simply due to the fact that the gut's good bacteria neutralize about 40 percent of the toxins we consume in our food, acting as a kind of satellite liver, of sorts. So, for deep and complete detoxification, you need at least a basic level of gut health. I understood this from the beginning.

What took me a little longer to grasp, however, was that gut dysfunction is at the root of most of today's health problems. But once I figured this out, everything started to fall into place, and I developed a sound, safe, and effective program for gut repair. This is what I present to you as *Clean Gut*.

My medical practice today is so much more rewarding because of the Clean Gut program, both for myself and my patients. I am no longer a diagnosis-making, prescription-writing machine. Before I even think of making a diagnosis, I immediately look for gut dysfunction. Often it is so obvious I don't even need any tests. After a twenty-one-day gut-repair program, so many of my patients' problems are completely gone. There's no need to order tests or prescribe pills. With an understanding of how the gut gets damaged, how gut dysfunction manifests as a multitude of seemingly unrelated and distant diseases, and, most importantly, how to help the body repair the gut, I was able to help many of my patients restore their true health. Such results led me to write this book. The Clean Gut program is a simple, lifesaving protocol designed to start you on the path to vibrant, lasting, prescription- and disease-free health.

This book is the culmination of the work and research I started when I set out to heal myself. I discovered that the gut is the root of health, and gut repair is the mother of preventive medicine. If your gut is healthy, there are almost no chronic diseases to prevent. For too long we have reacted to symptoms as our first steps in getting healthy. But with this new protocol, we offer a method to strike down disease before it takes hold. We no longer have to get sick to get healthy. With this new program we are able to transform our entire approach to health. Food is medicine, and the gut is the key to a long, vibrant life.

# CHAPTER THREE

# The Gut:
# Your Second Brain

Since I turned my attention to the gut, I have helped people resolve a varied list of symptoms and illnesses. From heart disease to autoimmune disorders to hormonal imbalances and infertility, understanding and repairing the gut is a pillar of my treatment approach. In my opinion, a clean gut means a clean bill of health. For true lifelong health, you must learn how to maintain a clean gut. The Clean Gut program provides you with everything you need to repair and sustain a healthy gut.

In the following pages, I will take you on a journey that will radically shift your understanding of the body and the root cause of disease. We will learn the ins and outs of how the gut is the root of our health and discover how gut dysfunction can cause chronic imbalances elsewhere in the body, which lead to a host of symptoms you may have never guessed were connected with it.

When I lived in India I heard many times about health and disease starting in the intestines. At the time, I had already come to understand that we indeed *are* what we *eat,* so I connected the dots and archived it as an interesting thought. Hippocrates expressed that "death lurks in the intestines" and that "bad digestion is the root of all evil." Later I recognized this as a profound concept, which had implications in every aspect of our lives, not only our physical bodies. Before you were born, all the building blocks to form the cells in your growing body were provided to you, in utero, by your mother, filtered and ready to use. This is the case until the umbilical cord is cut. At this point, your body immediately needs to acquire its many building blocks (nutrients) from the outside world, while making sure to keep out whatever it doesn't need and whatever is potentially harmful. Though it serves many minute and precise functions, the gut's most important—and difficult—function is to acquire the necessary building blocks for the body to build and run itself from the outside world, through food, while making sure that nothing foreign gets into the body, which could threaten its survival. Understanding how the gut achieves this miraculous feat, and how diet and lifestyle affect it, can save your life.

Your body has two brains: one in your head and one in your gut. When you have a thought, tiny sparks of electricity show up within the neurons in your head. The brain in your head is the hardware for your thoughts. But when you experience a "gut feeling," or intuition, the tiny sparks of electricity show up within the neurons in your second brain. While your first brain serves as your intellectual hardware, your second brain—the gut—is your spiritual and emotional GPS. Without it, you're lost.

The definition of the gut I provide in the following pages is my own creation. The reason I include the different parts of the gut under one name is because its functions are so intricately related and of such vital importance that thinking about them together will help you make better choices and decisions for your health. It will help you unlock the secret of super health. It will also help you understand what is wrong with medicine today and allow you to become your own doctor. Let's take a tour of this remarkable system.

The gut has four main parts:

- the digestive tube,

- the gut-associated lymphatic tissue,

- the intestinal flora, and

- the gut's nervous system.

An easy way to understand how your gut functions is to think of it in terms of a country. Every country has its own land and borders. Every country has in place specific infrastructure and communications systems. Every country has citizens and a department of homeland security.

Now, let's take a look at its different parts.


## The Digestive Tube

### Your Body's Busiest Border

Only three major organs come into physical contact with the outside world: your skin, your lungs, and your digestive tube.

It is easy to see how the skin is the border between the inside and outside of your body. Healthy skin is uninterrupted; most things bounce off it. The other two borders are more complicated. When you breathe, air enters your body. Even though oxygen comes in, it's outside of you until it passes into the lung's pulmonary capillaries and is carried away by red blood cells. The same is true for food and drink. When you swallow food, it disappears from your view and goes down the digestive tube. But it's technically "outside" of you until it is broken down and absorbed through the intestinal wall. Hence, the skin, the lungs, and the digestive tube encompass the three "borders" where the body draws a line between what is *inside* and what is *outside*.

Of these three organs, your digestive tube is the largest and busiest. The intestinal wall is also unique in that, unlike the lungs, it is constantly in touch with foreign stuff (food and drink, and all the chemicals we add to both) and foreign organisms (bacteria, yeast, parasites, and viruses, among others). And unlike the skin, which is designed to keep most things outside and let very few things pass through it, the intestinal wall is designed to absorb everything that is useful to your body.

The digestive tube measures between ten and fifteen feet, running from your mouth to your anus. Along this border, some of the most important functions for survival of your body are fulfilled, such as breaking down food (digestion), absorbing nutrients essential for life (absorption), eliminating waste from your blood circulation (elimination), and housing the intestinal flora. The digestive tube also functions as a structural framework within and around which the other parts of the gut—the gut-associated lymphatic tissue and nervous system—are organized.

## DIGESTION AND ABSORPTION: DISASSEMBLY AND IMPORT

As humans evolved, food was scarce. Our digestive tube adapted to make sure the cells of the intestinal walls would come in contact with food. This gave the body a better chance of absorbing whatever nutrients it could find. The body achieved this incredible task by creating folds and subfolds of the intestinal wall (villi and microvilli), which increased its contact surface area to—believe it or not—two hundred times the area of the skin covering your body.

The body acquires the nutrients necessary for its survival through digestion and absorption. Digestion is the process by which we break food into smaller pieces. It is done both mechanically (chewing) and chemically (digestive enzymes), and it involves different satellite organs, such as the salivary glands, liver, gallbladder, and pancreas. Absorption occurs once the broken-down food finds the cells of your intestinal wall (IW), the first layer of the body's cells to come in direct contact with the outside world. The cells of the IW let the smaller building blocks of food enter the body selectively through the cells or in between them, where they are tightly joined together in what are called "tight junctions." That is how nutrients get into the bloodstream.

## THE INTESTINAL WALL: CUSTOMS AND IMMIGRATION

The cells of the intestinal wall look very much like a brick wall. Each cell is closely attached to other cells by tight junctions. But these are highly intelligent bricks. They keep what is foreign to the body (undigested food and microorganisms) out while simultaneously letting in whatever the body needs—digested food. Cells of the intestinal wall release an antibacterial mucous coating that keeps bacteria at a distance from the cell membrane. They select what to let in and what to keep out, much like what happens at customs and immigration.

They normally let digested food in (as nutrients) and keep undigested food out of the bloodstream, as well as any foreign invaders (microorganisms), and even the good bacteria must be stopped from entering. For this reason, intestinal wall cells must always remain intact and their tight junctions must remain tight. A missing cell or a loosened junction would allow undigested food, and the good and bad bacteria inside the digestive tube, directly into your body. A discontinuation of intestinal wall cells or a loosening of the tight junctions—actual holes in the wall—leads to a condition called hyperpermeability, or leaky gut. This is the beginning of many illnesses.

Additionally, intestinal wall cells are in charge of exporting metabolic and other toxic waste outside the body into the digestive tube for elimination, joining along with whatever food the body didn't absorb. Most people think of their feces as whatever the body didn't want or need to absorb from the food they ate. But this is only half the story. The cells of the intestinal wall are capable of capturing other waste, such as mucus, fat, and toxins from our blood, and dumping it into the tube for elimination. This is the exact reverse of absorption. Even if you eat nothing, your body can form feces with this waste. I first noticed this during my first cleanse at We Care Spa. I ate nothing for ten days but I still produced stools. The average person usually passes remnants of food within two days, even if the system is backed up. Why, I wondered, was my body still passing waste? I later learned I was passing what is known as mucoid plaque. It was black and shaped like the foldings of the colon. Well into my detox, my body was starting to dig deep into my tissues for waste and dumping it into my digestive tube, where colonics then scraped it off like a dishwasher scrubbing at a dirty pot.

# The Gut-Associated Lymphatic Tissue (GALT)

## *Your Body's Department of Homeland Security*

As with any animal on the planet in competition with billions of other organisms for resources, our bodies have to function in the world as individual organisms. Big organisms like tigers and bears can kill us for dinner, but miniature or even microscopic organisms, such as viruses, parasites, and bacteria, can kill us just as readily. Big predators attack you from outside your body; microscopic ones kill you from the inside.

Foreign materials harmful to the body and foreign organisms must be kept outside. As I explained before, the first barrier that encounters anything foreign as it transits down the digestive tube is the intestinal wall. (The intestinal flora are actually the first barrier, but the bacteria are not considered your own cells.) In ideal circumstances, the IW cells with their tight junctions would be enough to fend off everything that is not completely digested food. However, some foreign materials (such as incompletely digested foods or toxic chemicals) or organisms may sometimes get through. This is where the body's gut-associated lymphatic tissue, or GALT, comes into play.

Your body's immune system works a lot like the U.S. Department of Homeland Security. It is in charge of detecting and destroying anything that comes into contact with your inside that is not recognized as simple nutrients or as a part of yourself. Your body's homeland security has many different divisions and uses an array of elaborate weapons, including immunoglobulins, or antibodies. Your immune system has B cells, T cells, mast cells, phagocytes, and many others, which all serve specific functions. Monocytes, for instance, attack viruses, while neutrophils attack bacteria. Eosinophils are involved in allergic-type reactions, and killer T cells attack cancerous cells, the body's terrorists. The different cells form different divisions, just as the United States employs the army, navy, CIA, and FBI in its War on Terror. Even though the cells of the immune system are located and circulate throughout the body, most troops and bases are deployed at the borders where the greatest danger lurks. This is why we find many immune-system cells right under the skin and around the lungs. But 80 percent of the body's security troops are deployed in the gut, right next to the border with the

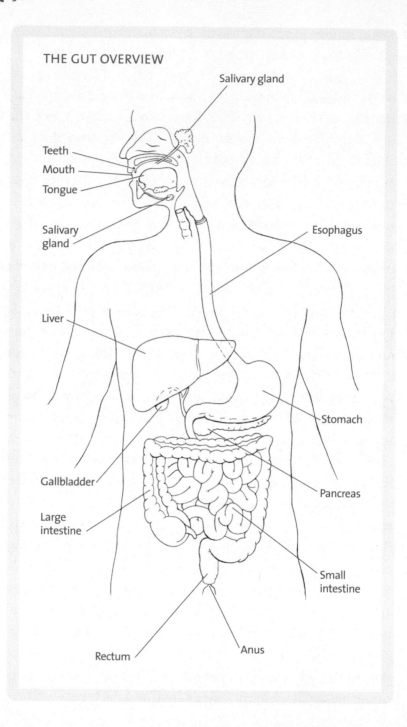

## THE GUT OVERVIEW

Salivary gland

Teeth

Mouth

Tongue

Salivary gland

Esophagus

Liver

Stomach

Gallbladder

Pancreas

Large intestine

Small intestine

Rectum

Anus

## THE HEALTHY GUT

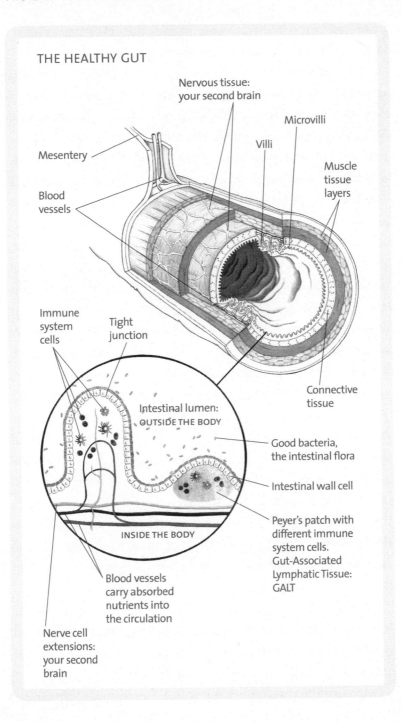

Nervous tissue:
your second brain

Microvilli

Villi

Mesentery

Muscle
tissue
layers

Blood
vessels

Immune
system
cells

Tight
junction

Connective
tissue

Intestinal lumen:
OUTSIDE THE BODY

Good bacteria,
the intestinal flora

Intestinal wall cell

Peyer's patch with
different immune
system cells.
Gut-Associated
Lymphatic Tissue:
GALT

INSIDE THE BODY

Blood vessels
carry absorbed
nutrients into
the circulation

Nerve cell
extensions:
your second
brain

most traffic: the intestinal wall. In fact, the GALT makes up the largest part of the body's entire immune system.

Our immune systems' cells are constantly scanning the environment to detect organisms and molecules that are foreign and hostile. It accomplishes this by recognizing surfaces. It helps to think of this system as similar to the scanning devices in stores. A simple scan of a tag will tell the retailer what a particular item is, how much it costs, and how many are left in stock. The body uses a code system called the HLA (human leukocyte antigen) system, which works in a similar fashion. It gives a code to all surfaces. Immune cells basically identify surfaces. Everything has a surface, whether it is your own cells, a microorganism, or a piece of food. When your immune system scans the interior surfaces of your body, it compares each to a list of approved codes, the ones it classifies as "self." If the immune system detects a surface with a threatening code, an antigen, it releases weapons and recruits other immune-system cells to attack the foreign surface as a way to defend you and survive.

When food is broken down, however, the individual surfaces of its building blocks are too small to be coded. As a result, the immune system interprets them as neutral. This is how you are able to absorb nutrients through your intestinal wall without alarming the immune system right underneath it. But if the surfaces of larger pieces of undigested food are presented to the immune system, it reads them as an antigen. Another way of saying this is that digested food is no longer antigenic; it no longer has a recognizable surface.

Here is where things can go wrong. Faced with a threat, the immune system launches a defense strategy that involves not only the immune cells in the gut, but also all the immune cells around the body. The body goes into full defense mode. It goes to war with the threatening surfaces, both animate (organisms) and inanimate (undigested foods and toxic chemicals). The immune system works best in certain conditions. For example, some of the immune system's divisions work best at a higher temperature. This is conveyed to the brain in the gut, which conserves heat by shutting down circulation to the skin to prevent heat loss as well as triggering muscle movements such as shivering, creating a fever in the process. A higher temperature when you are sick is not a mistake; it allows the immune system to perform more efficiently.

But the immune system requires a whole other set of conditions. This set of conditions is what we call inflammation. Often turned on by a dysfunction in the gut, inflammation is the body's best example of adapting and surviving. For millions of people around the planet, the gut is where systemic inflammation is born and from where it is sustained. Sustained systemic inflammation is what leads to many of the chronic diseases in the world today.

# The Intestinal Flora

### *Your Body's Tenants and Collaborators*

The giant folded area that lines the wall of your intestines is prime real estate for microorganisms to take up residence. They love it there. It's warm and cozy, humid, protected from the elements, and food falls from the skies. It is bacteria heaven. Throughout our natural evolution, we have become friendly with a number of them. We give them lodging and food. They pay us back by handling a heavy workload. And the gut is filled with these bacteria. In fact, there are more of them in a healthy gut than there are cells in the entire body. There are hundreds of different species of good bacteria. Altogether these bacteria can weigh as much as the liver, sometimes even more.

These microorganisms, called the intestinal flora, perform many important functions. Though the good bacteria of the intestinal flora don't share your DNA, they can—and should—be considered some of your own tissues, or even organs, given everything they do on your body's behalf. They are the first things other organisms encounter in the digestive tube, and they fight to protect their territory and prevent other organisms from taking hold. In this way, the intestinal flora helps the immune system fight invaders.

Even when there is no threat of invasion, the intestinal flora remains hard at work, constantly stimulating the GALT. Their effect on the GALT is known as immunomodulation. One of the most fascinating functions of the intestinal flora is their ability to regulate the immune system. Throughout the digestive tube different immune-system "stations" are located directly on the other side of the intestinal wall, opposite where the good bacteria settle. These good bacteria help keep the immune system in check. The immune system generally attacks bacteria, but it seems to have a truce with the bacteria of the intestinal flora, as long as they don't try to get into the bloodstream through the intestinal wall, which, as I mentioned previously, must always remain intact.

The presence of the gut's beneficial bacteria signals to the immune system that things are working well. Their presence also means that the climate in the gut is healthy. The immune system can't directly contact the intestinal flora, but one type of immune-system cell, called dendritic cells, sends filaments into the digestive tube through the intestinal wall to gather information of the conditions there and look for the presence of good bacteria. This is known as "snorkeling." The cellular activity of being constantly on the lookout for intestinal flora is what keeps the immune system awake and alert—ready for, but not engaged in, attack. The good bacteria regulate the immune system's baseline activity.

The intestinal flora does many other things as well. They digest part of our food for us. Certain nutrients, such as the B vitamins, have to be predigested by bacteria before the body can absorb them. Bacteria in general have different digestive systems from ours and can do certain chemical tricks with food that our bodies can't. Some of the digestive processes that the good bacteria perform are very useful to us. A healthy gut acts like a fermentation tank inside you. Because so many people's inner fermentation tanks are not populated with good bacteria, it is beneficial to consume fermented foods. "Fermented" really means that the food has already been digested by bacteria. In contrast, opportunistic bacteria and other organisms produce toxic waste from their digestion, such as flammable gases (methane) or neurotoxins, which paralyze the nerve–muscle terminals on your intestines and cause distended abdomens and constipation, among other things.

The intestinal flora is also a key contributor in detoxification, ridding the body of 40 percent of the toxins in food. In this sense, they serve as a satellite liver. Put another way, if the gut didn't have the intestinal flora, the liver would have to work almost twice as hard.

But our understanding of how many of which species of good bacteria and what segment of the digestive tube they should be in (small or large intestine) is pretty basic. And our understanding of how to repopulate the gut with good bacteria is even less complete. Nobody really knows what combination of species is the ideal one for an individual. What is unquestionable, however, is that they are beneficial.

We are just starting to fully understand what goes on in a healthy gut and, even more recently, how opportunistic microorganisms in our gut—such as viruses, parasites, yeast, and pathogenic bacteria—or the lack of good bacteria, are associated with many more problems than we ever thought. Look no further than the latest research in this fascinating area of study to understand the value of your intestinal flora, which is part of what's called the human microbiome. Just last year, for instance, studies emerged showing a strong connection between the state of our gut's ecosystem and cancer. The headline said it all: "What if a key factor ultimately behind a cancer was not a genetic defect but ecological?"

I believe there are many more discoveries to be made regarding how the intestinal flora communicates with cells in our bodies and helps us thrive and survive. But current research leaves no doubt that they have an essential role in our ability to thrive, stay healthy, adapt, and survive. Thinking of the intestinal flora as an integral part of our biology gives us more incentive to protect them and learn about them, as we do with every other organ in our bodies.

## The Gut's Nervous System

### Information, Communication, Coordination, and Much More

Within the walls of the digestive tube are many different layers of tissues. The intestinal wall, made of cells that absorb and eliminate food and waste, is the one layer in direct contact with the outside world. Around the intestinal wall is a layer of connective tissue, which holds in place the little blood vessels that collect whatever is absorbed. Another concentric layer of muscle cells squeezes the contents of the digestive tube forward. In between is a discontinuous layer of immune-system cells, organized mostly in bulks, or patches known as Peyer's patches. Tiny nerve filaments touch the intestinal wall cells, muscle cells, and immune cells that form the walls of the digestive tube, directing, regulating, modulating, and coordinating their functions. Muscle cells in the digestive tract, for instance, are responsible for peristalsis. The time of contraction of these cells, the strength, and the duration are all governed by these nerve filaments, which are extensions of neurons that live around the gut, essentially the brain in the gut.

The same is true with the intestinal-wall cells, the GALT cells, and the arteries and veins inside the gut. These nerve filaments, spread throughout the gut like a net, send and receive information to and from our gut neurons, which coordinate, modulate, and regulate all of them at the same time, continuously. In other words, the neurons in your gut orchestrate peristalsis and digestion, and modulate immunity and the hormonal system. Without them, the gut would cease to work.

As the tiny nerve filaments that innervate the neighboring cells join with one another, they form nerves, which are bundles of axons, extensions of the neurons that live in the gut. Amazingly, if you were to isolate these neurons and clump them all together, they would form a mass of neurons larger than the ones in your head. In fact, the brain in your gut is way more active in the production of neurotransmitters than the brain in your head. Serotonin, the neurotransmitter responsible for the feeling of happiness and well-being, is primarily manufactured in the gut—90 percent of it, in fact.

On top of all this activity, the brain in the gut helps run your intuition, communicating with you through feelings. These feelings are generated electrically inside your body by the neurons in your gut. That's why we call it a "gut feeling." It's a parallel, powerful sense of knowing. Listening to your gut is one of the most important lessons you can learn, which makes repairing and taking better care of it the most important thing for you to do.

• • •

Now that you have a better understanding of what the gut is and how it functions in a healthy body, I will tell you how it gets injured, little by little, on a daily basis. Even people who live very healthy lives are affected.

# CHAPTER FOUR

# How We Get Sick: Gut Dysfunction

So what exactly causes a breakdown in this elaborate, complex instrument we call the gut?

In my medical practice, I have never seen two people's health problems present in the same way. There's always a difference in how my patients experience disease, even if a disease is caused by exactly the same problem. People have very different tolerance levels for pain and other uncomfortable symptoms. We are also affected differently due to our varied fitness levels, nutritional status, support systems, and emotional states. It is the same when it comes to gut dysfunction. There are endless ways in which the gut gets injured, and at varying levels of severity. Understanding how each of the gut's four parts are affected independently is the foundation to realizing how distant and seemingly unrelated parts of our bodies can suffer combined dysfunctions.

In general terms, two parts of the gut—the intestinal flora and the intestinal wall—suffer first, while the other two—the immune system and the brain in the gut—respond to the situation with only one goal: survival.

## Intestinal Flora: Inner Annihilation

I begin with the intestinal flora because it is the first part of the gut that suffers the unnatural conditions of what is considered normal life for most of the planet's population. The body's intestinal flora, a key contributor in producing lasting health, is under attack from the moment of our birth. While giving birth is one of the most natural functions of all animals, the way humans do it has deviated substantially from the way Mother Nature intended—particularly in the United States, where pregnancy and birth are treated like a disease. It's dealt with in sterile hospital rooms. Mothers are hooked up with intravenous lines and set up in the strangest positions, which are designed more for the doctor's view and access than the mother's comfort and birthing process. Too many women are induced, which often leads to C-sections that would not have been necessary if the natural process of labor had been respected and allowed to proceed without disruption. A baby in the womb is sterile, but when passing through the birth canal, it is exposed to bacteria, mouth first. These bacteria are supposed to colonize the gut, nature's first vaccination of sorts. This does not happen during a C-Section. As part of this procedure, mothers are also injected with antibiotics, which end up affecting the baby's gut even more. Even when mothers deliver vaginally, induced labors cause more vaginal tears and episiotomies. In response, doctors prescribe antibiotics to prevent infection. And after that, women with mastitis—an infection in the tissue of the breast—

are often given antibiotics, which prevent good bacteria from colonizing in a newborn's gut.

Later, children are given antibiotics for every kind of infection—throat, ear, sinus, etc. In fact, because this antibiotic regime starts early, far too many of us have always lived with compromised intestinal flora and have never been truly healthy. I see more and more of this in my practice every year. It is my experience that chronically ill people, who often present with an elusive diagnosis, have a long history of consuming antibiotics. The earlier they started, the more complicated their symptoms are later in their lives and the harder it is for doctors to find a diagnosis. This is the case with several of my patients. They are surprised when I ask them if they were born by C-section, but many times they were. I call them the "C-section generation."

Health-related problems, however, often pop up regardless of the number of antibiotic courses taken during a lifetime. Some of my patients suffer greatly after a single course of antibiotics, even if the antibiotics were absolutely necessary. This is exactly what happened with Greg. He consulted me about symptoms that were not clear at all. Greg had frequent episodes of cold-like symptoms, which had been occurring regularly for over two years. The strange part was he never presented a fever or cough. He also suffered through bouts of depression, which affected him even though everything in his life was working well. When I asked Greg about his health history, he told me that he had had pneumonia two years earlier. Doctors—rightly—had prescribed a round of levaquin, a very strong antibiotic. The symptoms Greg was still experiencing led him to believe he'd never fully recovered from his infection. He was sure that the bacteria attacking his lungs had caused permanent damage. But a chest X-ray did not show any scarring. I explained to him that he had never recovered from the antibiotics prescribed to kill the pneumonia-causing bacteria. They saved his life by clearing the airways but ruined his life by killing the good bacteria in his gut. Greg's intestinal flora were decimated and his gut was compromised, which is why his cold-like symptoms persisted.

A compromised gut also explained his depression. His "second brain" was depleted and diverted, responding to the alarms coming from an immune system in full defense mode that had been triggered by dysbiosis and hyperpermeability, a result of the levaquin. By turning our attention to gut repair, specifically repopulating Greg's gut with good bacteria, my team and I were able to completely resolve his lingering symptoms.

Let me be clear here: I am not saying that we shouldn't use antibiotics when needed. Antibiotics saved my life when I was drowning with double pneumonia on my friend Richard's sofa. But we currently use antibiotics excessively and irresponsibly. We are wiping the population of good bacteria from the face of the earth, and we may not be able to live healthy lives without them. The medical profession—myself included—needs to be more prudent and vigilant about prescribing antibiotics so promptly.

This will only take us so far, however. There are other, more insidious antibiotics decimating our intestinal flora. These are found in our food. Some of the same antibiotics doctors prescribe to human patients are administered to livestock by the food industry. These antibiotics will kill your good bacteria as well. Now include the number of antibiotics the food industry adds to any processed food that comes in a box, jar, bag, tube, or bottle. Many chemicals are added to food during processing to kill any bacteria or funguses that would shorten a product's shelf life. The food industry calls them preservatives, but in essence they act as antibiotics. Other chemicals, such as coloring agents and texture, odor, and flavor chemicals, also make it hard for good bacteria to thrive. How else would something edible last for years without decomposing? Next time you shop the aisles of a supermarket, remember the longer the shelf life of what you are eating, the shorter yours will be.

The large amounts of food we eat, the excessive combinations, and the frequency with which we eat, even if we eat all organic foods, also play a role in the demise of intestinal flora. The combination of foods in our diets today is unprecedented. We mix many vegetables and fruits in one sitting. Many of these combinations are not natural and are often harmful to good bacteria, ultimately creating an environment in our gut in which opportunistic organisms thrive. Millions of people follow the media and the media doctors, who promote eating more fruits. But if you have an overgrowth of yeast, a frequent situation after antibiotic use, you may be throwing logs onto the fire. The sugar in fruit is on the list of a yeast's favorite desserts.

Opportunistic organisms are constantly traveling down the digestive tube. Despite their constant trips down there, they only take up residence when the good bacteria are not there to keep them out. Once introduced, these dangerous new occupants compete with us for valuable nutrients. They gorge on and thrive on all the garbage food we consume, which has no nutritional value whatsoever. Parasites then attack our weakened cells and tissues, essentially eating them for lunch, while viruses can take over your cells' DNA and make your own cells manufacture more viruses. This attack on the intestinal wall has several consequences. First, it prevents the body from absorbing valuable nutrients, which the body needs to manufacture things such as hormones, neurotransmitters, other cells, and that participate in the body's molecular activities. Plus, it exposes the immune system to a plethora of antigens (threatening surfaces), which forces the immune system into defense mode. The attack also depletes the second brain by forcing it to coordinate all the immune responses, which often prevents the body from completing many of its primary functions.

Take a look at B vitamins, for instance. These vitamins are the best example of the kinds of bacteria-dependent nutrients the body requires for, among other things, manufacturing red blood cells in the body's bone marrow, producing the chemical reactions required for detoxifying in the liver, and producing neurotransmitters inside our neurons. Without a healthy intestinal flora, the body can't fully absorb these essential B vitamins, which prevents the body from fully performing these crucial functions. Multiply this by a large number of bacteria-dependent nutrients and every other biochemical reaction in your body is affected. The consequences can be devastating. An unhealthy population of organisms in the gut is a condition known as dysbiosis, an inevitable consequence of the unnatural conditions in which we live and arguably the most common problem affecting people today. We are all walking around with some degree of dysbiosis. Dysbiosis is not a simple problem to diagnose and it can sometimes be very hard to correct.

The importance of a healthy intestinal flora cannot be overstated. Several studies suggest that changes in the composition of gut bacteria are linked to such varied diseases as obesity, inflammatory bowel disease, asthma, mental disorders, and many others. In the fall of 2012, for instance, scientists in China and Europe discovered that there is something recognizably different in the gut bacteria of people with type 2 diabetes. According to their research, people with type 2 diabetes have a more hostile bacterial environment in their guts. In other words, they have low levels of healthy bacteria and too many opportunistic pathogens.

When bugs enter the digestive tube, they are mostly acting independently. Even if there are billions of them, they are physically disconnected from one another. Once inside, however, they quickly understand that strength comes from community. Up to 80 percent of the organisms that cause problems in your gut, and the rest of your body, live in tight communities. But not just next to one another. They actually build—and live in— entire buildings, a condominium complex of millions of little organisms. When a few opportunistic organisms find themselves in the gut in close proximity to one another, they start producing and coating themselves with a mucous-like gelatin substance that fuses with the coating of the bacteria next to it. In medical terms, this combined coating is called biofilm, and it is the subject of intense research, largely because it makes organisms inside our bodies one thousand times more resistant to antibiotics. Here's how: Different species of bacteria, parasites, and candida (or yeast) can share a biofilm, which means it takes only a small presence of each to mobilize into a formidable army against the intestinal wall and immune system in the gut. This protective shield acts like a kind of bunker against other bugs, the body's immune system, and antibiotics. And it is a highly elaborate and intelligently designed bunker: it contains channels through which food and waste are moved.

On top of this, biofilm has the ability to sequester minerals and metals, especially heavy metals. These minerals and heavy metals include, respectively, calcium and iron, mercury and lead. With these minerals and metals, the biofilm becomes architecturally harder and therefore more resistant to elimination. For proper gut repair one must remove the organisms that shouldn't be there. There are natural weapons against them, most notably wormwood, artemisia, cloves, garlic, oregano oil, berberine, and mastic gum, among others. Pharmaceutical weapons include antibiotics, antifungals, and antiparasitics. But for any of these weapons to have a chance, the biofilm must first be dissolved or the organisms must be inhibited from manufacturing it. It may even be necessary to chelate the minerals and metals in it to soften it up. There are many ways to disassemble biofilm and many more under investigation. We will be using this knowledge during the Clean Gut program.

## The Intestinal Wall:
## Our Body's Achilles' Heel

As I said in the previous chapter, the intestinal wall serves three important functions: First, to digest foods and absorb nutrients, second, to shield the immune system from making contact with any foreign surfaces (antigens from undigested foods and organisms, both good and bad), and third, to get rid of waste from the body's bloodstream. When the intestinal wall is damaged, however, all these functions are impaired.

There are many ways in which the intestinal wall can be disrupted. Even though it is not a flat, smooth surface like the surface of your skin, the two are very similar. Your skin acts as a physical barrier between the outside and the inside of your body. It prevents foreign organisms and other materials from entering the body's circulation. This is a very important function; in fact, your survival depends on it. Foreign organisms can kill or cause severe injury once they enter the bloodstream, which is why, of course, you have to disinfect cuts. Organisms have a much better chance of sneaking inside the body when the skin is discontinued.

The same is true for the skin inside your intestinal tube. When these cells are damaged by opportunistic organisms, or when cells do not divide and replace those that have been damaged, holes form on the intestinal wall. Cells of the intestinal wall need certain building blocks in order to keep dividing and forming more cells to replace expired ones. Some of these building blocks, such as glutamine, are only readily available in a body that consumes a healthy diet and has a healthy gut to process and absorb these nutrients. When this is not the case, cells fail to form and cover the gaps. But even if there

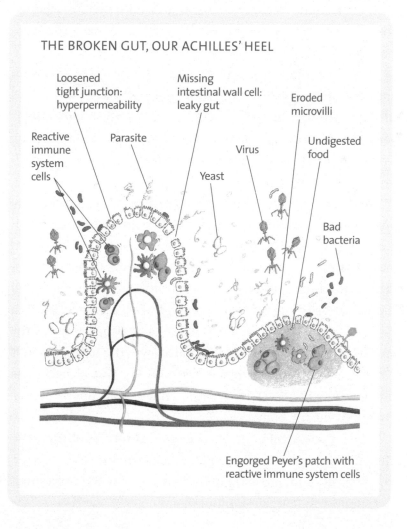

THE BROKEN GUT, OUR ACHILLES' HEEL

Loosened tight junction: hyperpermeability

Missing intestinal wall cell: leaky gut

Eroded microvilli

Reactive immune system cells

Parasite

Virus

Undigested food

Yeast

Bad bacteria

Engorged Peyer's patch with reactive immune system cells

are no missing bricks in the wall of the intestines, the tight junctions between them can loosen, which can also lead to increased permeability.

This is the anatomy of a leaky gut. And what does the gut leak, exactly? Two things: microorganisms and information. The information is in the surfaces of undigested food, organisms, and toxic molecules that the immune system is now exposed to due to the gaps in the intestinal wall. The immune system becomes directly exposed to incompletely digested foods, toxins, and a zoo of microorganisms it was never supposed to touch.

When the intestinal wall breaks down, its ability to absorb nutrients is diminished too. We are not really what we eat. We are what we absorb. Without vital nutrients, the body's important systems and functions slow down, which hinders the body's ability to eliminate waste from the circulating bloodstream, resulting in a toxic buildup.

The gut—the body's delicate, highly complex, and accurate instrument—is perfectly designed to live under natural conditions. The conditions we have created for ourselves, however, have started to break down the gut's intestinal flora and intestinal wall. As a result, the intestinal flora and intestinal wall are the first victims of our unnatural lives. Their deterioration is the beginning of disease for millions of people around the world. And, once they start to break down, the body responds by triggering specific survival mechanisms and an elaborate adaptation-compensation process, which ironically only further weakens the body.

This is our Achilles' Heel. The other two parts of the gut—the immune system and the brain in the gut—are left to adapt, compensate, and, most importantly, survive as their surrounding support system fails around them.

# The GALT: Homeland Security Confusion

When the intestinal flora and the intestinal wall deteriorate, the immune system in the gut is exposed to an unprecedented number of organisms, undigested foods, and toxic chemicals, all of whose surfaces the body identifies as foreign. As I already mentioned, this security breach calls the gut's immune system into action, immediately initiating a number of different responses. None of these responses are mistakes, but we experience them as such. These apparent mistakes can present as a nonspecific symptom, such as fatigue, which is often tricky to figure out the root cause of. This is especially true in the case of a hyperactive GALT. If you were able to isolate all the cells of the GALT and bulk them together, they would produce a mass larger than one of your quadriceps, the biggest muscles in your body. The function of a muscle is to contract and cause movement. That is what muscle cells do when they are at work—and they spend energy in the process. Imagine how exhausted you would feel if you had a disease that forced your quads to constantly contract. It would be easy to make the connection between a muscle at work and physical exhaustion. You would see and feel the muscle contract and relax, contract and relax.

A GALT in a constant state of attack—which is more or less the case for everyone today—is much like having a quad muscle in constant motion, though the cells of the GALT have a different function. Their work is silent in comparison to the contracting quadriceps, but, while there's no movement involved, the work is no less intense and no less taxing. When the cells of the GALT launch attacks, they use up invaluable resources and energy, just as you would expect of a battalion at war. The cells of the GALT manufacture antibodies and proliferate. They cause all kinds of chemical reactions, which cause corresponding effects in the rest of the body, such as when mast cells produce and release histamine, which in turn causes airway obstruction, vasodilation, mucus secretion, and itchiness, among other things. And someone may just feel exhausted, with no other symptom, unable to put his or her finger on what's wrong.

There are many ways in which the gut's immune system ends up causing havoc in cells, tissues, and organs all over the body. Many of the patients I encounter in my practice suffer from what seems to be a confusion of the immune system. In their mildest forms, these mechanisms end up causing specific symptoms, such as sneezing, itching, or coughing. These are mechanisms that are activated by the immune system in general to get rid of foreign invaders. Sneezing and coughing are attempts to get rid of airborne invaders, such as pollen or mites. So it seems logical that the immune system will try to get rid of them by any means necessary. Itching is a way the immune system tells you to scratch and get rid of something in the skin or mucous membranes, such as the eyelids and nose. I have seen many people, who are convinced they have seasonal allergies, get rid of their symptoms after gut repair. The pollen is still there, but after gut repair, they do not respond allergically.

Some people present with these same symptoms, but only when the GALT is triggered by certain foods. If the food in question triggers an immediate reaction, you may link it even with an itch or a cough. But the GALT has delayed mechanisms as well, which means that the itching and sneezing may begin up to seventy-two hours after the food was consumed. Sometimes, however, gut disruption presents as symptoms without an immediate, obvious function. This is what happens with skin rashes and lesions. When I see skin rashes that are not due to someone touching something and noticing a rash in the place of contact, or a rash caused by an insect bite, I look for gut invaders like parasites. Parasites do a number on the gut's immune system and they can present as the strangest of symptoms. In their more severe expressions, the mechanisms activated by the gut's immune system end up in total confusion, creating the most baffling of biological betrayals: an auto-immune disorder.

To make it easier for my patients to understand how this works, I use an admittedly simplistic analogy to describe in full the complexity of the body's immune system. But it's effective enough to give you a general understanding of how the immune system, in this case the GALT, functions and how it gets confused. Most people are familiar with LEGOs. On its own, each LEGO piece just looks like a basic generic shape. But when a few pieces are joined together, they can take the shape of anything—from something as basic as a building to something more complex, like an apple or a flower. If you showed a friend a combination of LEGOs, he or she would recognize immediately what you meant to build. But if you broke the combination of LEGOs back down to its individual blocks, your friend would never figure out what it had been a part of just a few minutes earlier. This is very similar to what happens with food at a cellular, molecular level. Whatever we eat is usually made of a combination of three types of main building blocks: proteins, carbohydrates, and fats. Mixed in with these are other nutrients, such as minerals and vitamins. When foods are broken down into peptides and amino acids (smaller protein building blocks), and simpler carbs and simpler fats, they can pass into the body through the intestinal wall and the tight junctions. Here is where the GALT waits to scan surfaces. As long as the food coming in is small, its surface remains neutral, as far as the GALT is concerned.

As mentioned previously, the body's immune system recognizes surfaces. Our cells have recognizable surfaces and so do microorganisms, undigested food, and foreign materials. Each surface has a code, and each cell of the immune system has a database of codes belonging to the surfaces that are accepted or recognized as "self." The immune system in the gut works by continuously scanning all surfaces that cross the intestinal wall. If a surface is not recognized as "self," an appropriate set of responses is initiated, the severity of which will match the gravity of the threat level of its code. The GALT then sends signals around the body—through the gut's brain and also through immune cells that leave the station in the gut and circulate throughout the body in our blood—to destroy anything with that surface code or anything with a similar surface code if the threat is considered grave. But sometimes the surfaces of our own cells and tissues fall into this "similar" category, so the immune system ends up attacking the body's own cells.

We currently understand quite a bit about surfaces and their codes and how the immune system reacts to them. But there is still much more to learn. The surface-code system in humans is known as the human leukocyte antigen (HLA) system, and these surfaces are part of the major histocompatibility complex (MHC). For instance, the autoimmune disease group spondyloarthropathies, which includes ankylosing spondylitis, reactive arthritis, and rheumatoid arthritis, among others, all share the involvement of a common surface code: HLA B27. Other autoimmune diseases, such as ulcerative colitis, Crohn's, iritis, and skin lesions, also feature the involvement of the HLA B27 surface code. It is not fully understood how the HLA B27 antigen affects the immune system. One theory is that many microorganisms in the gut, such as klebsiella, present the HLA B27 code. When the gut is hyperpermeable, the GALT is exposed to this surface, which triggers confusion in the immune system in such a way that it ends up attacking the joints and other organs.

This is what was happening to Magdalena and many of my other patients diagnosed with autoimmune diseases. Of all the illnesses that pervade modern society, autoimmune diseases continue to trouble and confuse doctors. Why does the body turn on itself? How can the immune system, which is perfectly designed to detect and deal with foreign invaders, suddenly think its own body is the enemy? It's as if the immune system gets confused over what's "self" and what's "non-self."

The type of autoimmune disease depends on what tissue, or what combination of organs, the immune system attacks. I always tell my patients it doesn't really matter what type of autoimmune disorder you have. What matters is how—or why—the immune system got confused. This confusion almost always occurs in the same place: the gut.

Another example of a confused immune system attacking its host is Hashimoto's thyroiditis. This often happens as a cross-reaction against gluten. In a gut with hyperpermeability that is exposed to gluten, the GALT mounts an attack against it. But certain surfaces of the thyroid system are very similar to the surfaces in gluten, so the thyroid ends up under attack.

This is as simplified an explanation as I can come up with, and it is still complicated. The detailed scientific explanation is even more confusing, sometimes to the autoimmune specialists themselves, the rheumatologists. Maybe because of all these difficult names and concepts, doctors feel less conflicted about simply scribbling out a prescription for steroids or chemotherapy.

Autoimmune diseases are on the rise, and every day I talk to someone who's been diagnosed with one and has started on steroids or chemotherapy to depress the immune system. In many cases, gut repair resolves the immune system's confusion and not only allows my patients to avoid such heavy medications, but also to see their health completely restored.

## The Second Brain: GPS Malfunction

Even under the most optimal circumstances the brain in the gut is super busy. It is constantly coordinating nearly every aspect of the gut's functions. Take, for instance, peristalsis—the contractions of the muscles within the intestinal tube—which allows food and waste products to move along the intestines. During peristalsis, the second brain sends signals to every muscle cell through nerve filaments, while also coordinating signals to and from the GALT. In this way the second brain not only modulates activity within the GALT's different bases, it also connects the GALT with the rest of the immune system throughout the body. Essentially, the gut's second brain serves as a communication infrastructure for the GALT.

At the same time, the gut's brain serves as an orchestrator of compensatory responses for the hormonal system. The most common example would be the stimulation of the adrenal glands to produce more cortisol as a basic primary response to stress. Once released, cortisol elevates the body's blood-sugar levels, which then requires the body to produce extra insulin.

Plus, the gut's brain is intimately involved in the process of digestion by regulating many of its aspects, such as squeezing the contents of the gall bladder into the small intestine at the right time. And it helps with hormone coordination and balance by communicating with glands and tissues. (I discuss more of the gut's brain functions in chapter 3, but it is impossible to describe them all.)

When there is dysbiosis and hyperpermeability, the brain in the gut diverts its attention to coordinate the responses of the GALT and compensates for many other imbalances that occur as a result of our Achilles' Heel injury. The second brain quickly becomes so busy coordinating these other "emergency" functions that the normal everyday functions also get affected. Peristalsis is one of the first to feel the pinch. Constipation is the most common symptom on the planet, even if most people suffering from it don't know it. One bowel movement a day is considered great by a lot of people, but it is really constipation's mildest expression.

Neurons communicate by manufacturing and releasing neurotransmitters. In order to manufacture them at the rate needed, nutrients have to be available. Some of the nutrients essential for neurotransmitter production are the first ones depleted in a dysbiotic and nonabsorbing gut, such as the B vitamins, magnesium, calcium, and potassium. This adds to the dysfunction of the second brain.

•  •  •

Now that we have a better understanding of why we get sick, we are going to take a closer look at how the most common chronic diseases in America—and the world—can be traced back to gut dysfunction. As will soon become even clearer, healing the gut is the single most important step we can take to ensure our lifelong health.

# CHAPTER FIVE

# Survival Disguised as Disease

One morning not too long ago, I was walking down my driveway and came across a most remarkable scene. Looking down, I saw a bamboo shoot sprouting up from the asphalt. The shoot had broken through the hard ground as if it were made of paper. This was a clear reminder to me that nature's strongest force is survival.

Our bodies are made with the same intelligence.

Have you ever been underwater a little longer than you are used to? Have you gotten to the point at which your body desperately needs a breath and starts to show signs of struggle? What comes after this point—the epic fight someone can put up in order to breathe again—is the classic example of all that is put into play by a human being's instinct for survival. On a cellular and molecular scale, this fight for survival is no less dramatic or intense. Inside our bodies, billions of cells undergo trillions of chemical reactions every second of every day to ensure our survival. Simply put, we are designed to survive.

If nature specifically designed our bodies to survive, why do we continue to get sick? The answer to this question is simple. We don't. Our bodies simply don't know how to get sick. What we call diseases are really just different forms of survival mechanisms. They are essentially the body's attempt to send a bamboo shoot through concrete.

The best-known survival mechanism is the fight-or-flight response. Putting up a fight or running for your life are two very different choices, but they have something in common. Both of them will be better achieved if the body is physiologically prepared for extraordinary efforts. To trigger this mechanism, your body enacts millions of molecular reactions and cellular behaviors that would take an encyclopedia to describe in full. Basically, though, your adrenal glands rapidly release adrenaline and noradrenaline. This, in turn, makes the muscle cells in your iris contract to dilate your pupils so you can see more clearly. It also makes your heart's sinus node cells—the heart's natural pacemaker—accelerate your pulse, which causes your blood pressure to rise. Your cells then burn glucose and oxygen at a much faster rate, and your nerve cells send electrical impulses faster too. A faster heart rate, higher blood pressure, and better vision will make either running from danger or fighting it more effective, thus maximizing your chances of survival.

The immune system functions in a similar way. It has many specific actions it can perform for different situations, with very different possible outcomes. Different divisions of the immune system's army are deployed for different threats. The white blood cells called neutrophils, for instance, attack bacteria, while monocytes, another type of white blood cell, go after viruses. When allergies flare up, eosinophils and mast cells are put to hard work, while phagocytes eat away ("phago," to eat) at dead cells and foreign objects.

While the immune system reacts differently to different threats, it does respond uniformly to most threats in one regard: inflammation. Inflammation is the name for a set of basic responses that establishes the inner conditions for the immune-system cells to get to work more effectively. Vasodilation and increased permeability of the blood vessels are two basic responses. These allow the migration of immune-system cells from inside the blood vessels into the area where they are most needed. In the midst of local inflammation, the temperature in the area rises, because immune-system cells function better in slightly higher temperatures. On a larger scale, this is why the body generates fevers during an increased demand for immune-system activity, such as during infections.

Local inflammation not only helps the immune system prepare for and wage battle against foreign invaders, it also establishes an inner weather system for the repair of the affected area, patching up of injured structures, forming scars, and eventually returning the damaged tissue to its original, pre-injury state. Localized inflammation is a perfect survival response, not the common underlying precursor condition now linked to most chronic diseases.

The real problem arises when inflammation becomes systemic. Systemic means "all around your system"—affecting your entire body. Systemic inflammation can linger undetected for years and lead to such chronic diseases as heart disease, cancer, diabetes, or any number of autoimmune diseases.

Systemic inflammation is hard to wrap one's mind around. The best way to picture it is to think about coagulation, inflammation's sister process. Coagulation, or blood clotting, is one of the most basic—but most important—survival mechanisms.

Here, briefly, is how coagulation works: Circulating through the bloodstream is a group of normally inactive proteins (clotting factors) and cells (platelets), which get activated when a blood vessel is injured to form a blood clot to stop the bleeding. This is a lifesaving, local survival mechanism. But what if this local process were to become systemic? What if all the blood inside your body clotted at once? You don't need to be a doctor to figure out what would happen, but just in case, I'll tell you: rapid death.

Inflammation is very similar to coagulation. Like the proteins in the coagulation system, the cells and molecules that make inflammation possible are also normally circulating through the bloodstream in an inactive state until they are needed. Whenever a tissue is damaged or invaded, inflammation is "activated" locally. But it can also be activated systemically. Once inflammation becomes systemic, it often wreaks havoc. In functional medicine, inflammation is often compared to a wildfire, relentlessly destroying everything in its path. Just as local inflammation heats up a troubled area, systemic inflammation literally burns you from the inside out.

But why does systemic inflammation happen? That's the million-dollar question. Why do so many people suffer from an inflammatory system that gets turned on systemically? This book is the solution and the answer to that question. Before chronic disease comes systemic inflammation. But before systemic inflammation comes gut dysfunction.

Although systemic inflammation affects different parts of the body, it almost always originates in the gut. What this means is that most of the symptoms and diseases that manifest in different parts of the body—from the heart to the joints—are really just complex consequences, or elaborate disguises, of one common problem: gut dysfunction.

In the rest of this chapter I will trace some of the most common chronic symptoms and diseases in the world today back to their origins in the gut.

# Heart Disease

The number-one killer in the United States is coronary artery disease, my bread and butter as a cardiologist. But I don't see it as a disease. To me, it is the best example of a survival mechanism turned deadly. And it can all start in the gut.

If the wall of an artery gets injured—a common occurrence when arteries are stretched because of stress and high blood pressure, or scratched by toxic and irritating molecules such as nicotine, trans fats, chlorine, additives, and oxidants—your body patches up fissures with cholesterol plaque, a kind of plaster, in an attempt to prevent the artery from further damage and bleeding. The cholesterol plaque also buys time for the cells in the arterial wall to divide and repair the injured area, covering it with new cells under the plaque. Eventually, once the irritating conditions subside, as happens in nature, the cholesterol plaque will be reabsorbed and the artery will look like new again. This is similar to what happens to an injury in your skin under a scab. New cells are growing and covering the area, so when the scab falls, your skin is as intact as it was before the injury. All of these crucial activities are triggered, stimulated, and sustained by local inflammation. Once the arterial wall is repaired, the body absorbs the cholesterol plaque because it's no longer needed.

This is a perfect survival mechanism. Unless the irritation continues, which it does—largely because of the unnatural conditions in which we live today. As a result, once the plaque-building mechanism is turned on, it never turns off. This leads to an overstimulated response driven by systemic inflammation, which is most often sustained due to gut dysfunction. Instead of getting reabsorbed, the plaque keeps getting built until it eventually blocks the flow of blood inside the artery. The plaque-building and plaque-reabsorbing functions work perfectly in natural conditions, where stressful circumstances and adverse metabolic conditions come and go. But the process becomes detrimental when the body is under constant duress due to systemic inflammation.

In the presence of systemic inflammation, arteries get irritated more often and more severely. Chronic, sustained systemic inflammation is already accepted as the most important risk factor for coronary artery disease. Statins such as Lipitor and Crestor prevent heart attacks largely because of their anti-inflammatory properties, not because they lower cholesterol, contrary to what many doctors and patients believe. Statins chemically block the cascade of reactions that activate systemic inflammation.

Once we popularly accept that chronic, sustained inflammation is mostly a survival response to a dysfunctional gut, we will be able to have a real impact on the biggest cause of suffering and death in America.

The connections between the heart and the gut don't stop there. The following is a connection that continues to boggle my mind. Most people know that if they experience pain on the left side of the chest, they may be having a heart attack and should strongly consider calling an ambulance or going to an emergency room. The problem is that heart attacks don't always cause chest pain. Sometimes a heart attack can present in atypical ways, confusing whoever is experiencing it into thinking something else is wrong. Often this proves fatal. The most common atypical presentation is indigestion. I don't yet fully understand it, but I cannot help but notice this paradox: the gut can be sick for years without showing any symptoms, but at the moment of a heart attack, when it is critical for us to know that the problem is located in the heart, the gut decides to play a trick and shows symptoms such as nausea and indigestion, which diverts our attention, often with deadly results. I wonder if the gut's symptoms are nothing but a desperate attempt by our intuition to relay the seriousness of the situation. A gut that triggers systemic inflammation will also have an overworked second brain, the instrument of intuition. Indigestion during a heart attack may just be the message of a distorted intuition instrument.

Coronary artery disease is not the only type of heart disease with strong connections to the gut. Bill was suffering from a completely different problem. At ninety-three, Bill was incredibly active and productive. His daily schedule alternated between journalistic jobs, book writing, swimming, walking, studying, and a busy social life. After noticing he was often short of breath, he visited several doctors and ended up in a top cardiologist's office. Several tests confirmed that his aortic valve—the valve at the origin of the aorta in the left ventricle of the heart—was significantly tighter than normal, a condition called aortic stenosis. This was the first time he heard anything was wrong with his heart. In less than a week, Bill was scheduled for an aortic valve replacement. Needless to say, the risk associated with this surgery is very high, but Bill's family and friends, and mostly his heart surgeon, scared him into agreeing to the surgery. Still, he desperately wanted a second opinion.

Because he had read *Clean,* he made an appointment to see me. I examined him at Lenox Hill Hospital, where I determined that his aortic valve was in fact narrow, moderately to severely so. But when he and I discussed his health history, I found out that his symptoms had started after a course of antibiotics doctors had prescribed for a urinary tract infection. In addition to shortness of breath, he felt bloated and gassy after meals. I immediately put him on a gut repair program before his surgery. To his surprise, but not mine, within ten days his shortness of breath was completely resolved, as was his bloating and gas. By the end of the three-week program, he felt well enough to cancel the surgery. His dysfunctional gut had been consuming way too much oxygen, which had led to his shortness of breath. Though the program couldn't expand his valve, it did correct his dysbiosis, made his intestinal wall less permeable, and calmed down his GALT. This freed up some much-needed oxygen and energy, which allowed him to continue his normal activities.

His heart valve had probably been narrow for decades, but it wasn't until his gut was damaged by antibiotics that he started experiencing shortness of breath. Aortic stenosis usually progresses and eventually needs a valve replacement. If he would have been much younger, I probably would have also insisted he get a new valve. But at ninety-three, open-heart surgery would have probably killed him or significantly reduced his quality of life for some time, perhaps the rest of his life. Gut repair, on the other hand, allowed Bill to avoid the surgery and, most importantly, completely reverse his symptoms.

## Cancer

Cancer is the name used for a number of different diseases with one thing in common: a group of cells have started to terrorize the body. These terrorist cells kill innocent cells around them by multiplying excessively, compressing neighboring tissues and organs, competing for nutrients, and releasing toxins into the circulation.

The current medical approach is to kill the terrorists with heavy artillery (chemotherapy) or cut them out with surgery. Chemotherapy mostly works by blocking the division of rapidly multiplying cells. Unfortunately, chemotherapy also kills healthy, noncancerous cells, which need to rapidly divide for the body to function. These include red blood cells in our bone marrow, cells in the immune system, reproductive cells, and cells in the intestinal wall, which allow for hyperpermeability and malabsorption. In other words, chemotherapy allows damaging substances into the bloodstream while simultaneously making it difficult for the body to gather nutrients from food.

Often chemotherapy kills the patient faster than the cancer. Strangely enough, the patient, the patient's family, and the doctors are all left with a sense of relief that they did everything they could. I felt this after cancer took my father's life. I went with him to his chemotherapy sessions and watched him waste away, piece by piece, until all that was left of him was skin and bones. I always wonder what would have happened if I had known then what I know now. If I had thought of cancer as a group of cells just trying to survive, would we have been able to save my father instead of killing him slowly with chemotherapy? What if instead of deploying chemical weapons of mass destruction we had tried to improve the poor internal conditions that had forced these cells to turn against my father in the first place? What if we had tried a holistic approach?

Like any good, law-abiding citizen, a healthy cell demands certain minimal requirements: a safe, clean place to live, food, education, and entertainment. And, just as in real life, bad things usually happen under bad conditions. When the streets are filthy, violent, and unsafe, or when the air is polluted, or a citizen doesn't have access to food, or foreign invaders constantly infiltrate a country's borders, a good citizen can turn to violence or extremism. But if you asked a terrorist, he or she will likely tell you that there is nothing wrong with them, that the system is unfair, that the conditions are intolerable. Or that the future is grim, that they're only doing what they have to do to survive, even if it means killing others. As terrible as this sounds, this is exactly what happens with cancerous cells.

Internally, the body's streets (arteries) are filthy (toxic), the atmosphere is polluted (by acidity), the food is bad (nutrient depleted), and foreign invaders regularly infiltrate the border (viruses, bacteria, parasites, and fungus are all associated with different cancers). Meanwhile, your body's homeland security forces fire dangerous weapons (systemic inflammation), which often turns normal citizens (healthy cells) into terrorists (cancer cells).

All of these terrorist-cell-promoting conditions—systemic inflammation, nutrient depletion, acidity, absorption of toxins, and an infiltration by invading organisms—are direct consequences of gut dysfunction.

I do not mean to oversimplify things. Cancer is the result of many factors. But even genetic factors are connected to the gut. Carrying the gene for a certain cancer does not guarantee that the cancer will develop. Genes can be turned on and off by the conditions in which the cell is living. Nutrigenomics is the science that studies how nutrients, a lack of nutrients, or toxic molecules absorbed from our food can activate a gene that was previously dormant. The conditions that turn cancer genes on, however, are mostly the result of gut dysfunction.

There are cancer-promoting toxins that do not enter through the gut. Toxic gases enter through the lungs; many toxins enter through the skin, and so do microorganisms. But they have a much higher chance of success in causing cancer in an existing climate of systemic inflammation. And this, for many people, is a survival mechanism triggered by gut dysfunction.

Any way you look at it, gut repair and maintaining a healthy gut will give you the best chance of restoring your health if you already have cancer. More importantly, if you are healthy, it will give you the best chance to prevent cancer altogether.

# Depression

Back in 1997, when I was diagnosed with depression, my psychiatrist told me that my brain was not producing enough serotonin. As he spoke, he pointed to his head, a gesture I perfectly understood as indicating where those lazy neurons were located. I didn't think about it again until much later. During my first functional medicine class in 2006 I was reminded that neurons in the gut manufacture most of the serotonin in a healthy body. My psychiatrist was wrong when he pointed at his head. He should have pointed at his gut. And I was wrong in thinking of those neurons as lazy. They were actually working harder than in normal circumstances, only they were either lacking the raw materials they needed or busy doing other work that took priority during a state of alarm, such as it happens when the gut is in dysfunction.

Serotonin is one of a number of different neurotransmitters—protein-based molecules that the neurons use to pass messages to one another. This is how neurons communicate. Serotonin is the neurotransmitter thought to be responsible for the feelings of happiness and well-being, and a lack of it is linked to depression. It requires specific nutrients for its synthesis, such as 5 HTP, vitamin B6, magnesium, and calcium. When the gut is dysfunctional and absorption is reduced, these invaluable nutrients are amongst the first to become scarce. Without them, neurons are unable to assemble enough serotonin.

An absorption problem is just one way in which gut dysfunction leads to reduced serotonin production and depression. Another is when the gut's second brain needs to turn its attention to other priorities. As discussed, the second brain is responsible for many things. During gut dysfunction, the second brain has to dedicate energy and resources to coordinate survival mechanisms, diverting its attention from the production of healthy levels of serotonin. Even with sufficient nutrients available, those nutrients will be utilized for the production of other neurotransmitters, such as dopamine, adrenaline, noradrenaline, and GABA (gamma-aminobutyric acid), all of which are needed for the neurons to coordinate the immune system's attacks and regulate all sorts of compensatory measures. Without the necessary manufacturing of serotonin, the body, mind, and spirit succumb to depression.

Serotonin not only affects our moods and happiness, it also affects functions in the gut, such as motility and digestion. In my case, the dysfunction in my second brain not only expressed itself as depression, but also as irritable bowel syndrome (IBS). This is why doctors often prescribe antidepressants for IBS, because antidepressants help relieve the symptoms of IBS.

Depression is a growing problem worldwide. More than 350 million people suffer from it globally, according to the World Health Organization; it's incredible to think that around 5 percent of the world's population suffers depression in the course of a year. There isn't a single area in the world where people are completely free from the disorder. Many experts believe that depression will soon outpace all other diseases as the leading cause of suffering in the world.

When I was depressed I felt lost, with a total lack of insight, and I was completely overwhelmed by doubt. I understand now that this was because my second brain, my instrument of intuition, was malfunctioning. The neurons in my gut were too busy helping my immune system fight the dysbiosis and the increased permeability of my digestive tube. After my gut restored itself to a healthy state, through gut repair and maintenance, that sense of being lost completely vanished and a strong sense of purpose was reborn. I decided I would tell everyone about it, and this is why I've written this book.

## Allergies

When I met my neighbor Tim, he insisted he was perfectly healthy. His only health concern was his mother's. To treat a rare case of iron-deficiency anemia, she had been getting blood transfusions and receiving iron intravenously for a few years. Tim wasn't happy with how his mother, a wonderful woman named Barbara, was being treated medically, so he asked me if I might know a different way—anything, he told me, to help her. After talking to Barbara about her health history and reviewing her lab reports, I decided to put her on a gut repair program.

As we were getting everything ready for the program, I noticed that Tim kept sneezing, scratching his nose, and rubbing his eyes. He told me he suffered from allergies every time the seasons changed. He blamed it on pollen. He didn't consider it a health problem. In his mind, it was just an environmental problem. He thought of himself as the picture of health and, except for the occasional respiratory infection for which he took antibiotics, he had no medical issues.

But when I explained to him that allergies most likely originate in his gut, he decided to join his mom on the program.

After only a few days his allergies had drastically improved, and by the end of the program they had completely disappeared, at a time of year when they were usually the strongest. In the three years since he finished the program, he hasn't had a single seasonal allergic episode.

Barbara experienced equally impressive results, if not more. After her gut repair program, coupled with a few months following the Clean Gut principles, she no longer needed transfusions. She looked and felt as if she had been reborn. Her doctors were amazed.

What we call allergies are really just an exaggerated response of the immune system to common and essentially mildly threatening foreign materials or invaders. The body comes into contact with a threatening surface and puts into motion certain mechanisms to try to get rid of the foreign material or invader: a sneeze, itch, cough, or tear to expel whatever it is the immune system is alarmed by. Regardless of where in the body an allergy manifests—in the lungs or on the skin, for instance—the confusion of the immune system can almost always be traced to gut dysfunction.

Like millions of other people who suffer from allergies, Tim thought the allergy (in his case, pollen) was the single problem. He had accepted the fact that he needed to take anti-allergy medication during pollen season. His theory went out the window as soon as he finished his gut repair program and his allergy to pollen went away. When he asked me how this happened, I simply smiled and said, "Tim, that is the way nature designed it. Your immune system at the border in the lungs was responding to pollen in an exaggerated way. Pollen only caused that reaction when meeting cells from the immune system in the lungs that were hypersensitive. They overresponded.

"The reason why gut repair resolved your symptoms is because it was the immune system in the gut causing a systemic state of alert, communicating with the immune-system cells in the lungs and making them overreact. Once the gut dysfunction was corrected, pollen never affected you in the same way again."

If, like Tim, people with seasonal allergies were to go through a gut repair program and continue to keep their guts clean, they would save themselves suffering and trillions of dollars in prescription and over-the-counter anti-allergy drugs every year.

## Autoimmune Diseases

If allergies are an exaggerated immune response due to gut dysfunction, autoimmune diseases are the total confusion of its troops.

Autoimmune diseases are those in which parts of the body are attacked by the body's own immune system. There is something very wrong with this situation. It is mind boggling, as if the director of the CIA were also its most feared terrorist. Who can people trust if they can't even trust their own security agents?

Of all the illnesses that pervade modern society, autoimmune diseases continue to trouble and confuse doctors. Why does the body turn on itself? How can the immune system, which is perfectly designed to detect and deal with foreign invaders, suddenly think its own body is the enemy?

I met Elise at a promotional talk I gave for my first book, *Clean,* at a health-food store in Manhattan. During the talk, I mentioned briefly how the confusion of the immune system starts in the gut. After the event, Elise told me her story. Diagnosed with lupus, she was already taking a heavy dose of painkillers and steroids for her joint pains. Neither medication was controlling her symptoms. Her rheumatologist wanted to start her on chemotherapy drugs. Elise told me she was excited about exploring the idea of a gut repair program. Though I never gave her a consultation, she ran with the idea. A few months later she contacted me on Facebook to tell me how she had put together her own gut repair program and was off all medications. Plus, she looked and felt years younger.

One of the ways in which the immune system ends up attacking the tissues of the body they should be defending is a phenomenon called cross-reactivity. When the gut's immune system detects certain threatening surfaces in the context of a leaky gut, it sends signals to the rest of the body's immune-system cells to attack the same surfaces elsewhere (in case the foreign invader has already gotten into the circulation). Some of these threatening surfaces may be very similar to surfaces of cells and molecules in your body, and the immune system attacks those as well. It cross-reacts against those surfaces. Such is the case during autoimmune thyroiditis, otherwise known as Hashimoto's. Certain people's immune systems respond to gluten exposure by producing antibodies against certain components of their thyroid systems (thyroglobulin antibodies and thyroid peroxidase antibodies), which cause thyroid dysfunction, or hypothyroidism, a very frequent diagnosis in America. This is a case of cross-reactivity between gluten and the thyroid system components.

Autoimmune disorders are almost always treated in the same way. After a round of painkillers and nonsteroidal anti-inflammatories (if the symptoms include pain), treatment continues with prednisone or some other steroid, which depresses the immune system and makes the attack on the tissues less intense, or cease altogether. This is like secretly adding Valium to the U.S. Army's drinking water. The troops will lose their edge; they'll be half-asleep. This is both good and bad. When the body's own troops are sleepy and drowsy because of medication, they simultaneously ease their attack on other threats, which makes people more likely to succumb to infections, develop cancers, plus a whole series of other negative side effects, including weight gain, water retention, and other hormone imbalances.

If steroid treatment is like adding Valium to the army's water, chemotherapy is like adding cyanide. Chemotherapy is quickly becoming a more common treatment for severe autoimmune diseases. And, as I mentioned, chemotherapy simply kills the immune system.

People suffering from autoimmune illnesses are relieved when they discover that the confusion of the immune system usually begins in the gut, but even more relieved by witnessing their symptoms disappear as their gut is restored to a healthy state.

Through gut repair I have helped patients like Elise, Magdalena, and many others reclaim their health and avoid dangerous medications for many different autoimmune diseases, such as Behçet's, lupus, ankylosis spondylitis, rheumatoid arthritis, Hashimoto's, and others.

## Back Pain

Back pain is the most common complaint and reason for medical consultations in the world. And gut dysfunction is often at the root of it. How are the two related? The explanation is so simple that it goes undetected, or isn't even considered, by most medical professionals today. It's simply a matter of space and pressure.

When the immune and nervous systems in the gut battle dysbiosis and hyperpermeability (leaky gut), blood flow increases to meet the higher oxygen and nutrient demands of
an army and communication network at war. As a result, the
entire gut becomes engorged. It expands and pushes the tissues and organs around it. It first pushes in the direction of the
abdominal wall, since there is less resistance on most people's
abdominal walls due to a general weakness of muscles there.
This causes the abdomen to protrude—the infamous belly so
many Americans are obsessed with. Take your shirt off and look
at yourself in the mirror standing sideways. If your abdomen
wall is showing a bump and you are not pregnant, your suffering gut may be pushing it forward. A lot of people think this is
just fat under the skin, but that is only part of the answer. Go to
any gym and look at the older bodybuilders. They have almost
no fat under their abdominal wall skin; you can actually see
the skin's veins in many (a sign of little fat under the skin), but
many of them still have a protruding, bloated belly.

The gut also pushes against neighboring abdominal organs,
including the kidneys, liver, ovaries, and uterus—causing dysfunctions of different degrees by reducing circulation in those
organs—and the vertebrae and its emerging nerves. Plus, it
pushes the diaphragm up, thus compressing the lungs in the
chest, which can cause shortness of breath.

To compensate for all this increased pressure, the body
readjusts its posture. The result is back pain in all of its varying
forms, each related to the specific ways in which an individual's body realigns to cope with how the engorged gut is affecting the different organs.

I myself suffered from debilitating back pain at different
times while I was sick. First, I saw back specialists and surgeons,
sports medicine doctors, and physical therapists. I underwent

a series of X-rays, a CT scan, and an MRI. There was no indication of a herniated disc, a common cause for back pain and sciatic nerve pain, nor was there any telling structural damage. All I was given were muscle relaxants, anti-inflammatories, and painkillers. Though I was grateful for them at the time, they did very little to quiet my back over the long term or to prevent recurring episodes.

One time, in India, I had an episode of intense back pain. Our team's chiropractor helped me adjust my posture. I also got hands-on healing, including Reiki, deep-tissue massage, and Rolfing. I tried to strengthen my core through yoga. I was also introduced to Dr. John Sarno's theories, which teach that back pain is mostly due to pent-up emotional disturbances. All of these strategies helped in one way or another, but my back just never felt right. Until a few years later, when I finally got my gut in order. That's when I made the connection between back pain and gut dysfunction. Reading the work of Dr. Xave Mayr confirmed my suspicions.

Millions of people take pain medications and undergo surgeries and extensive rehabilitation programs for back pain, the cause of so much suffering and prolonged absences from work. It turns out, though, that repairing the gut can put an end to many cases of back pain. A healthy gut means a healthy back.

# Infertility

A female body requires certain basic conditions to support the growth of a baby. Pregnancy in itself puts a female in a vulnerable state. A general sense of being safe, both at an individual and a cellular level, and an abundance of nutrients are prerequisites for reproduction. A sense of alarm in the GALT and second brain, triggered by dysbiosis and a leaky gut, is enough to prevent pregnancy. It creates an inner atmosphere that the body interprets as unsafe for pregnancy.

Today, millions of women live in a constant state of emotional and physical stress, as well as lack enough essential nutrients in their bodies. A consequence of this constant state of alarm is a higher level of cortisol production. Cortisol is the stress hormone; it helps the body adapt to stress. When one hormone goes up, a different one goes down to maintain homeostasis, the natural balance our bodies constantly work to achieve. The hormones that sustain survival mechanisms inhibit the hormones that create an adequate cellular environment for conception and gestation. This is the way nature designed it. After repairing the gut, and sustaining its health, a female body will be in much better condition to allow a pregnancy to happen.

## Gluten Sensitivity

Most people don't fully understand how much gluten affects human health. The list of syndromes and diseases associated with gluten sensitivity is endless. It affects all the body's systems: hematologic, reproductive, neurologic, endocrine, hepatic, rheumatologic, encephalopathic, dental, and cutaneous.

Gluten is associated with cancers of the mouth and throat, esophagus, small intestines, and lymph nodes. It is also associated with type 1 diabetes as well as thyroid disorders, such as Hashimoto's, the most commonly diagnosed thyroid dysfunction in America. Many patients achieve normalization of their thyroid function only after adopting a gluten-free diet.

Gluten sensitivity is also associated with other autoimmune diseases, such as Sjörgens syndrome and dermatitis herpetiformis. Hair loss, or autoimmune alopecia, is another presentation. It is also associated with depression, migraines, arthritis, fatigue, osteoporosis, and anemia, to name a few.

With so many scientifically proven or suspected connections to so many diseases, it is tragic that instead of removing gluten from our lives, here in America we put it in everything.

Gluten is a protein found in grains, such as wheat, rye, and barley. Its sticky, glue-like property, and many other properties, makes gluten especially useful to the food industry, which uses it in its products as a binder, filler, shaper, bulking agent, texturizer, and stabilizer. Gluten binds juices into food-like products for sweetening purposes. It prevents shrinkage of foods and moisture loss. It helps dissolve fats by emulsifying them into foods. It is added to beverages to provide "body." It retains water up to twice its weight, so it is added to meats and canned foods to increase profit per pound. It is also added to imitation cheeses for elasticity. It's in MSG (monosodium glutamate). It provides a glazing effect on the casings of hot dogs and sausages. It is present in malt used for the flavoring and coloring of most cereals, even ones marketed as gluten-free because they are made with grains that don't contain gluten. It is also used in the chemical formulas of ice cream, mayonnaise, corn meal, and instant coffee. Most importantly, it is in the comfort foods we love the most, such as bread, pizza, rolls, buns, pancakes, cakes, muffins, pasta, pies, and pastries.

Gluten is also used as an excipient in many pharmaceuticals and supplements.

It is almost impossible to escape gluten in America. Gluten is everywhere, and it can really do a number on the gut. To digest gluten, the cells of the intestinal wall produce a specific enzyme called transglutaminase. Transglutaminase breaks down gluten into its smaller building blocks, the peptides gliadin and glutenin. The cells of the intestinal wall then absorb these into circulation. The GALT scans their surfaces, as it does with all things absorbed, in search of threatening surface codes. For reasons that only nature understands, the surface of the glutenin peptide is not coded as threatening, but gliadin is in people with a genetic predisposition. T cells in the GALT will mediate the production of gliadin antibodies. These same antibodies, however, often attack the intestinal wall's natural transglutaminase enzyme, essentially tearing apart the intestinal wall, piece by piece. This shrinks and erodes the villi and microvilli, the finger-like tendrils in the small intestine that maximize its surface area; this results in an inability of the small intestine to absorb any nutrients at all. In its most severe expression, this is known as celiac disease, which presents as weight loss, diarrhea, bloating, abdominal pain, and an overall failure to thrive.

This severe form of presentation is relatively rare, but for every person diagnosed with celiac disease there are an estimated eight others whose symptoms are atypical and therefore much harder to diagnose. Analysis of data has shown that when people are finally diagnosed, they have been suffering for an average of ten years.

Celiac disease and its milder and atypical presentations are the result of an autoimmune mechanism initiated by the GALT upon detecting the surface of gliadin. Glutenin can also trigger a series of reactions, which result in destruction of the intestinal wall and gut dysfunction, but not by glutenin's surface being recognized as threatening. Glutenin stimulates the immune system to release interleukin-15, one of the immune system's most lethal weapons, which it employs in the detection and elimination of cancerous cells. Interleukin-15 eats up the intestinal wall, which leads to abnormalities in absorption and permeability. It is just a chemical property of glutenin.

Today, gluten sensitivity is considered a common systemic autoimmune disease. Knowledge of the different ways in which the disease presents and the different organs it can affect is just starting to emerge in the medical community, thanks in large part to the hard work of the Institute for Functional Medicine. Avoiding gluten is especially important during gut repair programs, but for many it is important to avoid it permanently.

• • •

The list of disguised gut dysfunction does not stop here; I could write an entire book on gut dysfunction and its related illnesses. The connection between gut dysfunction and chronic disease should now be very clear. Yet gut health continues to be ignored when it comes to treatment options. The current medical approach to our long-term healthcare is frankly unsustainable. Disease is winning. But we can change this equation. We can restore the gut and reclaim both our day-to-day and long-term health. In the next few chapters, I detail the Clean Gut program and provide us all a much needed and newfound path to living disease-free.

# CHAPTER SIX

# The Clean Gut Program

## Why Gut Repair?

Gastrointestinal disorders are among the most common reasons for seeking medical care. They can range from mild symptoms—bloating, cramping, gas, constipation, abdominal distention, discomfort, or simple difficult digestion—to life-threatening conditions like bleeding, obstruction, infection, or severe inflammation. The different diagnoses made in these cases include, but are not limited to, peptic ulcers, gastroesophageal reflux, gastritis, diverticulitis, cholecystitis, appendicitis, ulcerative colitis, Crohn's disease, and irritable bowel syndrome.

Many of the symptoms that these gut disorders cause are clearly related to the gut because they are localized there. But as we have discovered there is ample evidence that many other diseases seemingly disconnected to the gut are also either rooted in gut dysfunction or highly affected by it. These include cancer, heart disease, autoimmune disorders, depression, allergies, and skin disorders, among others. In my medical practice, it has been my experience that addressing gut repair first can resolve or dramatically improve most of the chronic diseases affecting people today as well as many acute problems.

The weakest point in our biology in general is the gut, which is why I call it the body's Achilles' Heel. It is the part of the body that suffers the most damage from the unnatural way of life we have created. You can be sure that if you currently live in a modern city, you have some level of gut damage, which causes a degree of gut dysfunction and can lead to a whole spectrum of symptoms and diseases. Even if you are not currently experiencing any symptoms, gut damage today is what breeds diseases in the future.

This idea is easier to understand if we think of inflammation. Most people who educate themselves on health matters are aware that inflammation can go unnoticed and lead to chronic diseases after long periods of dormancy. Blood tests, such as a C-reactive protein (CRP) test or a test of the erythrocyte sedimentation rate (ESR), can detect inflammation even before any symptoms are noted. Even the most traditional of Western allopathic doctors, who are finally catching up to the dangers of inflammation, have started ordering these tests routinely. That doesn't mean they know what to do with the results, however. Most doctors I meet treat inflammation as the disease itself and deploy all sorts of anti-inflammatory weapons, from natural fish oils to synthetic drugs such as statins. They still consider these measures "preventive" since inflammation precedes a chronic disease.

But this approach is still a pill for an ill. If we focus on gut repair instead, we resolve systemic inflammation at its source. This is why periodic gut repair is the best preventive medicine of all. I strongly believe that periodic measures toward gut repair have prevented problems in many of my patients, to the point of even slowing the inevitable process of aging.

Whenever I encounter people who are in great health for long periods of time, I ask them a lot of questions. Intentionally or unintentionally, I find that all of them have incorporated practices and principles of gut repair into their lifestyle. Here, I give you the road map to longevity and vibrant health. The Clean Gut program is your ticket to a disease-free journey with an upgrade to first class.

## The Clean Gut Program Overview

During the first phase of the Clean Gut program, for twenty-one days you will drink a liquid breakfast and enjoy delicious lunch and dinner meals from the Clean Gut diet. You will also take recommended supplements and practice specific activities that will enhance the process of gut repair.

After the gut repair process—in phase two of the program—you will reintroduce foods into your diet over the course of a week, which will allow you to identify the foods that do not promote long-term gut health. In the process, you will also create your own dietary blueprint to fit your specific needs and lifestyle.

## Phase One: Gut Repair
## (Twenty-One Days)

### *The Four Pillars of Gut Repair*
The Clean Gut program is based on the four pillars of gut repair, known in functional medicine as the four Rs: Remove, Replace, Reinoculate, and Repair.

**REMOVE**

This aspect of the program is about removing from the gut anything that poses an obstacle to the gut's optimal function. This could be toxic organisms, such as viruses, bacteria, yeast, or parasites. It can also be toxic molecules, most of which come in our food and drink, such as preservatives, additives, hormones, antibiotics, heavy metals, and chlorine, to name a few.

Even food without toxic molecules can still trigger toxic reactions in the gut, such as dairy, gluten, and grains, among many others. One way in which food affects the body negatively is by generating allergic reactions. More and more people are becoming aware of the potential allergenic effects of food, and more and more doctors are starting to order blood and skin provocation tests to detect these food allergies. Blood tests typically measure immunoglobulins (antibodies) against different kinds of food. Food not only affects the body by activating responses of the allergic type, but it can also activate other mechanisms in the body, such as autoimmune responses, or create other adverse conditions, such as acidity, mucus formation, bloating, or constipation.

The Clean Gut program aims to eliminate in one stroke all the foods that prevent or delay gut repair, including some that feed the toxic organisms, which need removal as well. The conditions created by the Clean Gut program—and the program's supplements—remove many of the most common organisms that lead to dysbiosis, including bad bacteria, mild to moderate levels of yeast overgrowth, and even some very mild viral and parasite invasions. (See page 110 in the "The Clean Gut Program's Spectrum of Intensity" section for a list of conditions the program will not fully eliminate.) Since a vast majority of invading organisms organize themselves in protective-shielding biofilms, the Clean Gut program is designed to dissolve these as well, a prerequisite to correcting dysbiosis in many cases. (See pages 132–133 for a list of which supplement does what.) There are other factors that go beyond the contents of the digestive tube that the Clean Gut program does not specifically address but are worth giving attention to, such as removing oneself from stressful situations and unhealthy relationships, and even removing negative feelings and thoughts. Additionally, reducing exposure to toxic chemicals in city water is an important part of the Remove pillar. City-supplied water in most cities in America is loaded with toxic chemicals, from chlorine and fluoride to all kinds of medications and remnants of toilet paper. One of the most important things we can do for our long-term health is filter all water in our homes, especially in the kitchen. I am lucky to have found William Wendling, who continuously teaches me about water filtration. He is a fountain of information and tools. Check his work at www.oxygenozone.com.

## REPLACE

The Clean Gut program replaces invaluable nutrients in the body. These include magnesium and other minerals, vitamins, good proteins, good fats, fiber, and complex carbs. The program creates conditions in the gut that allow for better absorption of these nutrients, while its recipes and supplements are designed to flood the body with all the nutrients the body needs to function at its peak, most notably digestive enzymes such as proteases, lipases, amylases, and cellulases, among others, which aid in the process of gut repair.

## REINOCULATE

Removing the "bad" organisms from the gut is only half the battle. We also have to replant and feed the gut's intestinal flora, the body's good bacteria. This is done with the probiotics and prebiotics included in the Clean Gut program. The most beneficial species of good bacteria include lactobacillus acidophilus, lactobacillus thermophilous, lactobacillus bulgaris, lactobacillus casei, saccharomyces boulardii, and bifidobacterium longum, though there are many others. The program includes multiple species of good bacteria, all of which feature a high enough quantity of beneficial organisms to maximize the chances of a robust colonization of good bacteria within the gut.

## REPAIR

The intestinal mucosa, the cells that form the intestinal wall, are most in need of architectural repair. Their division and growth—and the tightening of their junctions with neighboring cells to patch up a leaky gut and hyperpermeability—require certain conditions and essential nutrients, which the Clean Gut program creates and provides respectively.

*"The past couple of weeks everyone in my family has been sick with fever, sore throat, and very bad sinus congestion. On Tuesday afternoon, I had a fever, chills, and swollen glands. I was sure I had succumbed to the virus. I awoke Wednesday morning not feeling 100 percent but not feeling as bad as the night before. I had heavy bags under my eyes, and some sinus pressure, but overall I thought there was a potential to kick this. Today—absolutely nothing! No bags, no pressure, fever and swollen glands are gone. And . . . [I received] comments from people on how well I look. There is no way I would have fought this type of virus before the Clean Gut program!"*

—Holly

## *The Clean Gut Diet*

The Clean Gut diet focuses on eating easily digestible, low-sugar foods while avoiding the kinds of food that lead to gut dysfunction. We've included a list of basic principles you'll be following on the program, a quick guide, which tells you the key categories of foods to eat and to avoid, and a food list, which gives you a full breakdown of the Clean Gut diet.

### BASIC PRINCIPLES

The 80-20 rule is a simple way to remind yourself which foods to eat and how much.

> Fill 80 percent of your plate with greens and vegetables (raw, steamed, baked, cooked) and 20 percent with protein and good fats (meat, fish, avocado, etc.). There is no need to count calories. This is a visual process; just look at your plate and fill 80 percent of it with greens and veggies and the remaining 20 percent with your protein and good fats.

> Stop eating when you are 80 percent full. This will help your body digest more easily. Absorption and digestion are just as important as the types of food you eat. This will take time to master, but giving it attention during the program will go a long way toward making it a part of your daily practice.

### COMBINE MINDFULLY

For better digestion, follow these basic rules when combining food:

> Pair vegetables and greens with animal protein (fish, meat, eggs).

Pair vegetables and greens with vegetable protein (lentils).

Don't pair animal protein and vegetable protein. (For example, don't eat chicken and quinoa; instead, eat chicken and veggies or quinoa and veggies.)

QUICK REFERENCE GUIDE*

Here is a quick snapshot of the major foods you'll eat and avoid on the program. Some foods, like beans and certain fruits, have been excluded from the Clean Gut diet because they are difficult to digest or high in sugar, even though they are a staple of most healthy diets. Once you've completed the Clean Gut program, feel free to reintroduce them into your regular diet.

| EAT | DON'T EAT |
| --- | --- |
| Greens and fresh vegetables | Gluten |
| Lentils, quinoa* | Dairy |
| Wild fish | Processed sugar |
| Grass-fed meats | Alcohol |
| Organic or pasture-raised eggs | Caffeine |
| Fermented foods (kimchi, sauerkraut) | Beans |
| | Rice |
| Nuts, seeds, and nut butters** | Soy |
| Avocado | Potatoes |
| Coconut | Corn |
| Fresh and frozen berries | Almost all fruits |

*Go easy on these, only a side serving a day
**Go easy on nuts, only a handful a day

---

*The Clean Gut diet grew out of the elimination diet in *Clean*. However, we've made significant changes to maximize gut repair.

## CLEAN GUT DIET FOOD LIST

### EAT

*Vegetables:* whole vegetables (broccoli, kale, chard, etc.) raw, steamed, sautéed, juiced, or roasted; all leafy greens; squash; tomatoes; and sea vegetables.

*Fruit:* only fresh and frozen berries, lemons, and limes.

*Dairy Substitutes and Eggs:* eggs; hemp and nut milks (almond, hazelnut, walnut, etc.); coconut milk; and coconut oil or butter.

*Grains:* quinoa; go easy on quinoa.

*Meat and Fish:* fresh or water-packed cold-water fish (trout, salmon, halibut, tuna, mackerel, sardines, pike, kippers, etc.), wild game (rabbit, pheasant, bison, venison, elk, etc.), lamb, duck, organic chicken and turkey, and small amounts of grass-fed beef.

*Vegetable Proteins:* split peas, bee pollen, spirulina, and blue-green algae.

*Nuts and Seeds:* most nuts and seeds, hemp, sesame, and sunflower seeds; pecans, almonds, walnuts, cashews, pistachios, macadamia nuts, and Brazil nuts; and nut and seed butters (almond, tahini, etc.).

*Fats and Oils:* avocado and coconut; extra-virgin olive, flax, safflower, sesame, almond, sunflower, walnut, pumpkin, and coconut oils.

*Drinks:* filtered, seltzer, and mineral waters; green, white, and herbal teas; yerba maté; coconut water; and green juices.

*Sweeteners:* stevia, xylitol, and Lakanto.

*Condiments:* vinegar, all spices, all herbs, sea salt, black pepper, carob, raw chocolate (dairy- and sugar-free), stone-ground mustard, miso, coconut liquid aminos, wheat-free tamari, and nama shoyu.

### DON'T EAT

*Vegetables:* corn, beets, potatoes, sweet potatoes, yams, and creamed vegetables.

*Fruit:* all fruits and fruit juices except berries.

*Dairy:* milk, cheese, cottage cheese, cream, yogurt, butter, ice cream, and nondairy creamers.

*Grains:* rice, wheat, millet, amaranth, buckwheat, barley, spelt, kamut, rye, triticale, and oats (even gluten-free).

*Meat and Fish:* factory-farmed meats, cold cuts, canned meats, and frankfurters (hot dogs).

*Vegetable Proteins:* all beans, lentils, and soybean products, including soy sauce and soybean oil in processed foods.

*Nuts and Seeds:* peanuts and peanut butter.

*Fats and Oils:* butter, margarine, shortening, processed oils, canola oil, salad dressings, mayonnaise, and spreads.

*Drinks:* alcohol, coffee, caffeinated beverages, soda pop, soft drinks, and fruit juices.

*Sweeteners:* refined sugar, white and brown sugars, maple syrup, high-fructose corn syrup, evaporated cane juice, Splenda, Equal, Sweet'N Low, juice concentrates, agave nectar, and honey.

*Condiments:* regular chocolate (with dairy and sugar), ketchup, relish, chutney, traditional soy sauce, barbecue sauce, teriyaki sauce, and breath mints.

To see what a day following the Clean Gut diet looks like, visit cleangut.com.

## Supplement Recommendations

Supplements are an integral part of the Clean Gut program. They are essential for all aspects of the four Rs.

Here is a list of supplements you'll need to participate in the program. They are available online or at your local health-food store.

Visit cleangut.com to see recommended supplements.

**HERBAL ANTIMICROBIAL**
**(one recommended serving, taken twice a day)**
Preferably a formula with Berberine, such as Berberine HCL 400 mg or Berberine Sulfate 400 mg.

**SACCHAROMYCES BOULARDII**
**(one recommended serving, taken twice a day)**
At least 5 billion count live organisms per serving.

**MULTIPLE-STRAIN PROBIOTIC**
**(50 billion bacterial count, taken twice a day)**
It is best to pick up a probiotic at your local health food store. Choose one that has the lactobacillus acidophilus strain and other strains such as Bifidobacterium longum, lactobacillus rhamnosus, Bifidobacterium bifidum.

**MAGNESIUM**
**(250 milligrams, off citrate or glycinate, taken once a day)**
You can find this supplement in capsule or powdered form.

**MULTIPLE DIGESTIVE ENZYMES**
**(one recommended serving, taken three times a day)**
A product that contains multiple digestive enzymes such as protease, amylase, lipase.

**BIOFILM-DISSOLVING SUPPLEMENT SUCH AS MONOLAURIN (600 milligrams per serving, to be taken twice daily)**

Monolaurin is a powerful antibiofilm dissolver and antimicrobial made from concentrated lauric acid found in coconut. It is sold in capsule form.

**B VITAMIN COMPLEX CONTAINING B12, B6, B5, AND OTHERS (minimum doses per serving are 500 mcg for B12, 50 mg for B6, and 100 mg for B5, to be taken three times daily)**

A quality B vitamin complex will help support balanced moods, healthy energy levels, and the nervous and immune systems.

| SUPPLEMENT CHECKLIST | PURCHASED? |
|---|---|
| Herbal antimicrobial | |
| Saccharomyces boulardii | |
| Multiple-strain probiotic | |
| Magnesium | |
| Multiple digestive enzymes | |
| Monolaurin | |
| B vitamin complex | |

Visit cleangut.com to see the supplement brands I recommend.

## Clean Gut Daily Protocol

This is the basic protocol to be followed for the duration of the program.

**FIRST THING IN THE MORNING**

A glass of water with half a squeezed lemon.

**BREAKFAST**

A green shake plus supplements. See "Recipes" (page 151); any of the shakes described there are good for breakfast. Ideally, you will vary them, but you can benefit from any of them, even if you drink the same shake every day.

*Supplements:*

- 1 herbal antimicrobial
- 1 saccharomyces boulardii
- 1 multiple-strain probiotic
- 1 multiple digestive enzyme
- 1 monolaurin
- 1 B vitamin complex

**LUNCH (Main Meal of the Day)**

A soup, entrée-size salad, and/or entrée from the "Recipes" section (page 158–209) or a meal made up of Clean Gut Diet-approved foods (page 95).

*Supplements:*

- 1 multiple digestive enzyme
- 1 B vitamin complex

**DINNER**

An entrée-size salad from the "Recipes" section (page 203); or any salad variation made up of Clean Gut Diet-approved foods, plus supplements. After dinner take a ten-minute walk. Even a short walk helps aid digestion, encourages bowel movements, reduces stress, and provides a moment to reflect on the day.

*Supplements:*

- 1 herbal antimicrobial
- 1 saccharomyces boulardii
- 1 multiple-strain probiotic
- 1 multiple digestive enzyme
- 1 monolaurin
- 1 B vitamin complex

**IMMEDIATELY BEFORE BED**

- magnesium

*"I've noticed a remarkable thing in the past few days. I have pretty severe ADD. One of the symptoms is a high level of anxiety and a racy brain. I'm almost always with some kind of stimulation: the TV, a book, net surfing, computer solitaire. The distraction of the stimulation eases the anxiety. But I've noticed in the last few days that I'm preferring the quiet. I'm choosing to keep the TV and music off. My focus is better. I'm more present for my son. I have so many friends who think this way of eating is deprivational and punishing. If eating this way offers me clear skin, consistent energy, deep sleep, loss of anxiety, and a focused mind, I would say it's well worth the extra effort."*

—Anita

# Phase Two: Reintroduction (Seven Days)

The reintroduction process is the last stage of the Clean Gut program (days 22 to 28). While staying on the Clean Gut diet, reintroduce gluten and dairy over seven days. The purpose of the process is to identify your toxic triggers. Toxic triggers are foods that cause inflammation, acidity, irritation, or indigestion. They can also cause allergic reactions and food sensitivities, which are not allergic in nature, but negative nonetheless. Without realizing it, you most likely consumed some toxic triggers before starting the gut repair program.

The goal of the seven-day testing period is to discover your specific toxic triggers. If you simply go back to your normal diet immediately after the program, without knowing what your toxic triggers are, you may feel "off" without knowing why.

Before we begin, however, let's take a closer look at different types of toxic triggers.

## Toxic Triggers

Toxic triggers are foods that may taste great but more often than not leave you feeling terrible. They can cause mood swings, indigestion, bloating, and fatigue. They may also trigger an autoimmune reaction. Toxic triggers often promote the proliferation of unhealthy organisms inside the gut. The most common toxic triggers are gluten, dairy, processed sugar, caffeine, and alcohol. Getting clear on your toxic triggers will undoubtedly improve your health and prevent your mood, weight, and energy from yo-yoing up and down. During your reintroduction process you'll focus on the two most common toxic triggers: gluten and dairy.

I can't stress enough how important it is to identify your toxic triggers. It really is the foundation of building a clean gut and living clean for life.

## Getting Started

Getting started with the reintroduction process is easy. Now that you've finished your gut repair program, you will begin to eat three solid meals a day from the Clean Gut diet. Over the next seven days, you'll reintroduce gluten and dairy to find out how these two toxic triggers affect you. Understanding your relationship with these two foods is one of the best things you can do to improve your long-term health.

> "I'm feeling really amazing being on the gut program. Curious to see how I continue on this after our thirty days. I want to continue being vegan and gluten-free. I'm feeling really great. My first week was an adjustment but now I feel like my body and mind are really flowing with it all. My experience was great! I really enjoyed the program. I started to introduce foods again that were on the "Don't Eat" list, and I could immediately feel the difference. I want to continue with my gut program."
>
> —Dalila

## *The Reintroduction Process*

The reintroduction process will take seven days.

| | |
|---|---|
| Day 22 | Gluten |
| Day 23 | Gluten |
| Day 24 | Clean Gut Diet only |
| Day 25 | Clean Gut Diet Only |
| Day 26 | Dairy |
| Day 27 | Dairy |
| Day 28 | Reflect |

### STEP ONE: REINTRODUCE GLUTEN

On the first and second day of your reintroduction week, you'll add gluten back into your diet. Eat gluten two to three times a day for the first two days, and note how you feel over the next forty-eight hours. You'll continue to eat meals from the Clean Gut diet; the only difference is that you'll gradually add gluten to determine if gluten is one of your toxic triggers.

Reintroducing gluten by itself is simple. Try adding just bread to your breakfast and then some pasta for lunch or dinner. Don't include any dairy or other excluded items yet. The goal is to isolate one excluded food at a time to determine if it is one of your toxic triggers. A bowl of cereal, for example, wouldn't be the best choice because it includes dairy and wheat. If you have cereal in the morning and notice that it doesn't sit well with you, it won't be clear whether it was the dairy or the wheat that acted as a toxic trigger.

Karen finished the Clean Gut program's initial repair phase and felt fantastic. She had lost seven pounds and slept better and more soundly than ever before. She felt a greater sense of clarity. Her skin looked vibrant.

Then, she moved on to the reintroduction phase. Karen had always thought she didn't have a problem with wheat, especially whole grain, but she was surprised to learn how gluten truly affected her. She had a very strong reaction when she reintroduced whole-grain bread and pasta back into her diet. She recorded in her food journal that she felt bloated and constipated, and experienced mood changes. Sometimes she even felt irritable and short-tempered. Though Karen didn't enjoy the process, she was relieved to figure out that wheat was a toxic trigger for her. The real question was what to do with this information.

Because Karen's reaction to gluten was so strong, she decided to remove it almost entirely from her diet. She upgraded certain foods and evolved others. Instead of eating traditional wheat pasta twice a week, for instance, she opted for gluten-free pasta made from brown rice. Instead of having a side of bread with her

### STEP TWO: KEEP A JOURNAL

Use a journal to record any reactions you might have to gluten. This may include bloating, skin breakouts, a fogginess of the mind, or constipation. Not everyone will react to gluten in the same way. Some people may notice their reactions immediately. Others might notice their reactions the next day. That's why it's important to test gluten over the course of two days.

The following questions will help guide you:

Did anything happen shortly after eating it, such as a runny nose or mucus in the throat (typical of milk), or fatigue, bloating, or a headache (typical of wheat)?

soup or a slice of toast in the morning, she enjoyed a side salad and a bigger omelet for breakfast. She frequented gluten-free recipe blogs and got creative with meals to keep them interesting. Although she did consume gluten a couple of times over the next few months, mostly at social occasions, she was later able to recognize how gluten affected her because her symptoms returned.

Karen's reaction to dairy was a little milder. After reintroducing dairy into her diet, she noticed that the only reaction she experienced was minor congestion. After the reintroduction process was complete, Karen made the decision to cut her dairy intake. And when she did have dairy, she focused on primarily eating hormone-free and organic dairy. Every so often, when Karen didn't feel 100 percent, she removed dairy completely for a few days just to make sure she wasn't reacting to it.

Even though this whole process was a big shift for Karen initially, she was willing to take it one day at a time, because she'd never felt better than when she was on the Clean Gut program and she wanted to maintain those results as best she could.

How were your energy levels? A bowl of wheat pasta at night, for example, may make you feel tired immediately after eating it or upon waking the next morning.

How were your bowel movements the day after eating gluten? Were they as frequent and as easy as they were during your gut program?

Did you sleep poorly? Did you have intense dreams or nightmares? Did you wake up in the middle of the night?

How did you feel emotionally the next day? Were you angry, moody, or irritable?

### STEP THREE: EAT FROM THE CLEAN GUT DIET

After you have reintroduced gluten—and documented its effects on you—return to eating three meals a day exclusively from the Clean Gut diet for the next two days. Returning to the Clean Gut diet sets you up for testing the next possible toxic trigger: dairy. Think of these two days as a palate cleanser, like smelling coffee beans in between samples of different fragrances.

### STEP FOUR: REINTRODUCE DAIRY

For the next two days, you'll reintroduce dairy into your diet. Eat dairy two to three times a day for two days, and then note what happens over the next forty-eight hours. Once again, you'll still be eating meals from the Clean Gut diet; the only difference is that you'll be adding dairy to see if it is one of your toxic triggers. Try drinking a glass of milk in the morning, for instance, and adding a few pieces of cheese to your lunch or dinner. Today, dairy is included in many different foods. It's important to avoid having dairy in combination with other excluded foods. Stay away from cereal, ice cream, or baked goods, all of which contain processed sugar, gluten, or preservatives, among other excluded foods. If you have ice cream, for example, and it causes a reaction, you'll have no idea which excluded ingredient was the cause.

### STEP FIVE: REVIEW YOUR JOURNAL

Now that you've tested both gluten and dairy, review your journal. Your goal here is to figure out whether gluten and/or dairy are your toxic triggers. The way we determine this is by examining how strong your reaction was to each one.

Let's review the possible reactions you may have had during the previous few days:

*No Reaction:* "I felt fine. I didn't notice any changes in mood. I felt energized and awake. I felt good."

*Mild Reaction:* "I felt bloated and gassy. I felt tired. I felt dehydrated. I felt itchy. I felt uncomfortable. My sleep was off. I felt foggy."

*Strong Reaction:* "I felt sick. I developed a lot of mucus. I had a strong headache. I was flushed. I was very constipated. I developed a rash. I had trouble sleeping. I felt cold- or flu-like symptoms. I developed diarrhea. I became very angry or upset."

Take a look at your journal. What types of reactions did you have to gluten or dairy? If you had a mild or strong reaction to one or both of these foods, chances are they are toxic triggers for you. Discovering that either gluten or dairy is a toxic trigger is an amazing find. Before completing the Clean Gut program, these foods affected you without you knowing it. Not anymore.

So now what? What do you do once you've gotten clear on the fact that gluten or dairy is a toxic trigger? It's time to create a game plan.

## STEP SIX: REMOVE AND ROTATE

Creating a game plan starts when you decide whether you need to either remove or rotate your toxic triggers. Let's take a look at both options.

### Remove

If you had a strong negative reaction to a toxic trigger, your body was telling you that it's important to eliminate this food from your diet completely for a period of time. Removing a favorite food from your diet can be challenging, but the long-term benefits outweigh the short-term gratification. Many people continue to become healthier simply by removing their key toxic triggers.

*Rotate*

If your reaction to a toxic trigger is mild but still noticeable, it may not be necessary to eliminate that food forever. However, you will benefit greatly from reducing your exposure to it. Rotate your choice of foods in such a way that you don't eat the irritating ones more than once a week.

> *"I used to have water retention and watery eyes before the program but I have not had that since day three of the program. I notice a better immune system and have not caught colds others have had that I would normally have. My concentration and mood has been better. Although I am not overweight, I did lose five pounds that I had put on in the last year. Great experience!"*
>
> —Tiffany

## Advanced Reintroduction: Going Beyond Gluten and Dairy

During the seven-day reintroduction process we focused on gluten and dairy, the two most common toxic triggers. But these aren't the only ones. For those of you who want to explore other potential toxic triggers, or are already clear on your relationship with gluten and dairy, begin testing the foods listed below. Follow the same process as before—eat the potential toxic trigger two to three times a day for two days. Then take a two-day break before you start a new food item.

As you discovered during the gut program, the type of food you eat matters a lot. Your choice of food is often the difference between feeling energized and alive and feeling tired and sick. While this process does take time, it is one of the most revealing and inexpensive ways to determine what foods will promote your highest level of long-term health.

Here is a list of the most common toxic triggers:

- corn
- eggs
- soy
- red meat
- nightshade vegetables (potatoes, tomatoes, peppers, eggplant)

# The Big Three:
# Processed Sugar, Caffeine, and Alcohol

I call processed sugar, caffeine, and alcohol the Big Three. They are toxic triggers, but they are different from gluten and dairy. Gluten and dairy are often considered health foods, but no one would encourage us to eat more of the Big Three to get healthy.

Still, most of us either do consume them or will consume them in the future. So, it's important to understand our relationship with them.

## *Removing Dependency*

It's common for people to become dependent on processed sugar, caffeine, and alcohol. Dependency can be physical and psychological. It is the feeling that we have to have it or the sensation of feeling off when we don't. Removing dependency allows us to enjoy these items from time to time without significant health consequences. I approach dependency on the Big Three in two ways: crowd out and pulse out.

## CROWD OUT

We need to eat good quantities of healthy food each day. When we don't, we feel anxious or irritable. This is when cravings occur. This is also the reason why most diets fail. Diets focus on eating less rather than adding healthy food. When you focus on including a lot of delicious, nutrient-rich, whole foods into your diet you end up "crowding out" the junk.

For example, if you want to reduce your cravings for processed sugar or sugary foods, you need to eat enough low-sugar foods throughout the day. If you don't eat enough of the good stuff, cravings arise quickly, especially if you are tired. It's best not to depend on willpower alone to deal with these cravings. Crowding out the junk is one of the simplest tools to leverage your own willpower and remove dependency.

> *"I feel awesome! For me, cutting out sugar was a huge change. I have a true understanding now of how foods affect how I feel, and I don't need nearly as much food as I think I do. I felt so much more energy during the program and felt free from not having to rely on alcohol, caffeine, and sugar. I also lost five pounds and am now in the 'normal' BMI range. Thank you for offering this program!"*
>
> —Esther

## PULSE OUT

To pulse out means to remove something from your diet for a period of time. Doing this allows you to feel the true effects of whatever item you are testing. The reintroduction process is an example of pulsing that occurs at the end of your Clean Gut program.

If you want to remain free from dependency on the Big Three, it's important to take breaks from them. Pulse out coffee, sugar, and alcohol. This could be for one week or one month—

what matters most is that you give yourself a break from them so that you can remind yourself of their true effects when you add them back in.

Here is a simple example: During the Clean Gut program, you removed alcohol for three weeks. As a result, your body is now able to give you a reliable response about the true effects of alcohol on your system. You want to reproduce this effect by pulsing out alcohol throughout the year, not just during the gut program. If you don't take a break every so often, you can easily forget the effect this item has on your health. Pulsing out is something you do repeatedly over time to remind yourself of how these foods actually affect you. When you are clear about the effects of an item and are reminded again every so often, you learn how much of the Big Three your system can tolerate and how to enjoy them without negative health consequences.

## The Bigger Picture

There is no need to be a purist for the rest of your life, if you enjoy the foods I mentioned previously. Have them and enjoy them, bringing your awareness fully to the present moment with each bite or sip. There's often nothing worse for digestion than guilt. What's most important is that you notice the strong connection between what you eat and how you feel. Take time to explore this process. Your relationship with food wasn't created overnight, and it won't be reset overnight either.

There are thousands of theories about diet, lifestyle, and stress management. On top of that, it seems everyone has an opinion on how you should live and what you should eat. But nothing is more reliable than your firsthand experience. Completing the reintroduction process empowers you to listen to your body and make your own decisions about which foods work best for you.

# The Clean Gut Program's Spectrum of Intensity

Depending on the degree of gut dysfunction, your gut repair will require a specific degree of intensity. The Clean Gut program addresses the issues that end up creating mild to moderate dysbiosis and hyperpermeability. The vast majority of people fall into these two categories. (More severe cases will require additional measures and tools not included in this program.)

The severity of gut dysfunction varies for four reasons:

1. The toxic organisms present may be beyond what the Clean Gut program is designed to remove. These include severe yeast overgrowth, parasites, viruses, and certain bad bacteria, such as salmonella, Escherichia coli (E. coli), or Clostridium difficile (C. difficile).

2. Other influences may cause a severe leaky gut, such as heavy-metal toxicity or full-blown autoimmune-induced inflammation, including Crohn's disease and ulcerative colitis, which impair the regeneration of the cells of the intestinal wall.

3. Mechanical obstructions may interfere, such as constrictions, scarring, or an impacted, dilated colon.

4. Diverticulitis may be present, with pockets of infection.

Of these four reasons, only the final two require immediate medical attention and surgery. Antibiotics, anti-inflammatories, steroids, and chemotherapy agents may be lifesaving or allow someone to function again by suppressing debilitating and dangerous symptoms. If you know or suspect that you suffer from either of these conditions, do not try a gut repair program on your own at this time. If you do not want to go down the traditional route of prescriptions and medications, consult with a functional medicine doctor, who knows when to use pharmaceuticals and surgery, when to embark on an intense gut repair program, when and how to transition from one to the other, and how to combine all the different approaches when needed.

The first two examples, though probably already present in the gut, often remain concealed. As a result, they are rarely diagnosed. When they are diagnosed, doctors usually treat only their symptoms, not gut dysfunction. Think about parasite invasions. Patients with parasites, who suffer immensely for long periods of time, are often misdiagnosed and given treatments that only alleviate their symptoms. The parasites, therefore, continue to wreak havoc inside the gut.

Celine consulted me because she was experiencing severe panic attacks. On a couple of occasions, her anxiety was so high she took herself to the emergency room. But her electrocardiogram always showed only a slightly accelerated heart rate, and her blood tests always came back normal, though her white blood cells were slightly elevated. The doctor on duty each time she visited the emergency room attributed this to her panic attacks. She also had been previously diagnosed with endometriosis, which showed up as severe menstrual cramping, bloating, gas, diarrhea, and acne on her forty-three-year-old face.

When she came to see me, she had already seen many doctors and had countless tests performed. I discovered that all her problems had started after she received IVF hormone treatments to get pregnant with her second child. As I often do after hearing such complicated cases, with so many symptoms involving so many organs and systems, I asked her to collect all the test results she had amassed over the past three years. I told her to start the Clean Gut program in the meantime, knowing that it would take her at least three weeks to gather the information from so many different doctors' offices.

Celine completed the program before she was able to get all her records. All her symptoms had cleared up during the program, except for her acne, which had actually worsened in the second week of the program and persisted.

Just as I had done before with many other patients whose skin remained blotchy and irritated despite a drastic change in diet, I ordered stool tests for Celine, to check for parasites. Bingo. I found three different types of parasites and a severe overgrowth of yeast. I told her to continue with the Clean Gut program, and I put her on a round of nitazoxanide and fluconazole, pharmaceuticals for yeast and parasites, as well as a series of specific antiparasite and antiyeast herbs, including wormwood, oregano oil, and walnut hull, among others. I also prescribed extra intestinal-wall-repair supplements, such as aloe vera, colostrum, licorice root, and others, as well as lactoferrin, serrapeptase, and nattokinase to dissolve possibly stronger biofilms. Last, but not least, I started Celine on a combination of ashwaghanda and shatavari ayurvedic herbs, which are incredibly effective in balancing female sex hormones. Celine stayed on this strict, intense, and complicated program for about three months, save for the prescription medications, which lasted only ten days. Three months was all it took to reverse three years of constant suffering and periodic panic attacks. To this day, Celine's symptoms have stayed away completely. All of them.

Celine's health issues were not resolved by the initial twenty-one-day Clean Gut program, but without it she would never have found out about her parasites and severe yeast overgrowth, which ultimately lead to the resolution of her symptoms. It is not uncommon to find that parasites and yeasts are behind such complex conditions, which in Celine's case had eluded gastroenterologists, cardiologists, ob-gyns, and endocrinologists, each of whom had come up with different diagnoses.

Not only did the Clean Gut program uncover Celine's secret companions, it was also the basic protocol upon which I added different "treatment modules" to the program—one module for parasites, another for yeast, and another for hormonal balance.

I have had patients who, despite completing the Clean Gut program, did not improve from certain allergic and auto-immune conditions, and in these cases, further investigation lead to the discovery of toxic mercury, lead, or arsenic levels, sometimes revealing all three were present. In such cases, gut repair and the resulting health issues did not resolve until the heavy metals were chelated, either orally or with intravenous chelation.

The Clean Gut program will most likely be all the majority of people need to experience what it is like to have a clean gut. For others, the program will be the first step in uncovering a more deeply rooted problem. If you find yourself here, it is important to seek out a functional medicine doctor who can help you dig deeper. Either way, the program is the first step toward lasting health for everyone.

# CHAPTER SEVEN

# Guiding Principles for Living Clean for Life

The Clean and Clean Gut programs I developed did not emerge out of theoretical interest or a knee-jerk reaction to do things differently than what I was taught in medical school. My motivation came from a search for nonprescription solutions to my own health issues. Once I experienced the healing capabilities of cleansing and gut repair, my goal has been to help as many people as possible reclaim their health.

When it comes to transferring a three-week program into a sustained lifestyle, I, like so many, have had some difficulty. Long-term change is vital to make certain you don't slip back into old ways and undo all the good work. This type of change is very achievable, but it brings with it many obstacles. In order to overcome these, what is needed are experienced guides who know how to help us navigate all the possible bumps along this journey. For years, the Clean community has been a vibrant hub of knowledge, dialogue, and resources empowering tens of thousands to discover their path to lasting health. And that is why I have asked two Clean team members, Dhru Purohit and John Rosania, to share their knowledge and proven principles. These seven principles that Dhru and John are excited to offer are some of the simplest and clearest ways I've seen to help guide you to making healthy choices long term.

• • •

Most people conclude the Clean Gut program feeling great, with an increase in energy, improved digestion, heightened mental clarity, and usually some weight loss. The most common question we hear after people have completed it is, "I feel great, but how do I maintain the results?" The answer to this question is very straightforward: follow the guiding principles and practice what they teach.

The guiding principles are a collection of big ideas that will help you navigate the world of wellness after you've completed the program. They are not hard and fast rules. They are simply the principles that produce the best—and longest lasting—results for our team and our community. These principles work best when you personalize them, by taking what works for you and modifying what doesn't.

Today, we face more choices about our health than ever before. Not only do we have to navigate a landscape of unhealthy food choices, we also have to sort through loads of conflicting health information. To deal with this information overload, simple principles can help us cut through the noise of conflicting opinion. Principles help to shape how we make decisions each day. They also give us a foundation to turn to when we are unsure what to do next.

Let's take a closer look at our guiding principles:

What Not to Eat

What to Eat

How to Eat

Supplement Right

Understand the Psychology of Clean Living

Move and Chill

Create Community

## What Not to Eat

As we mentioned before, most people conclude the gut pro-gram feeling great. But they don't always know exactly why they feel so good. The supplements and the shakes play a major role, but the primary reason people feel good is because for twenty-one days straight they've stayed away from the most common toxic triggers—foods that cause indigestion, inflam-mation, bloating, fatigue, and, if consumed over long peri-ods of time, minor sicknesses, full-blown diseases, and major health challenges. Toxic triggers are making us sicker, fatter, and unhealthier than ever before.

Think of toxic triggers as little tacks, like the ones we use to pin up posters and calendars. Now imagine one day you left a few tacks in your back pocket and forgot they were there. You go about your day and eventually sit down to get some work done. Immediately you feel a sharp pain in your rear end. What would you do? Naturally you'd stand up and remove the tacks. What if instead of getting up and removing the tacks you con-tinued to sit on them in spite of the pain? And when the pain got much worse you simply took a painkiller to deal with it.

That sounds crazy, doesn't it? And yet that's exactly what is happening today. The only difference is that we're not sitting on our toxic triggers; we are eating them. And we're trying all sorts of pills, procedures, and roundabout fixes to deal with the symptoms that toxic triggers are creating, instead of dealing with the root cause. If you want to thrive, you have to remove the tacks. You have to know what not to eat and make the connection between the food you eat and how it makes you feel. Toxic triggers prevent your body from functioning properly. When you remove them, you remove the irritation they cause and stop the survival mechanisms your body puts into motion to deal with them.

Even if you eat healthy after completing the Clean Gut program, you still could have major health issues return, because your diet includes one or a few toxic triggers you may not know about. Finding your toxic triggers is the most important first step in living clean for life. That's why "What Not to Eat" is our first guiding principle.

When we understand what not to eat, our lives change. Health becomes less of a mystery and many health issues that may have affected us for years sometimes just disappear. Energy levels increase and our minds get clearer. Sleep gets deeper, more restful. Allergy symptoms are reduced or are completely relieved. The skin gets smoother and a certain glow emerges. The benefits transcend the body. People are more productive in their work, more attentive to their families, and more agile during exercise. Some people get a surge of courage, which allows them to overcome obstacles that have limited them for decades.

How is this possible? How could simply avoiding certain foods affect our long-term health so much? As the author Michael Pollan taught us in his book *The Omnivore's Dilemma*, our food and the way we eat has changed more in the last fifty years than in the last five thousand. All these changes mean that we're eating in a way that's significantly different from our ancestors. High-fructose corn syrup, corn-fed factory-farmed meat, preservatives, genetically modified wheat, and hormone-injected dairy are all examples of foods that have never been consumed in the quantities and combinations that we're consuming them in now.

Our food is changing, often for the worse, and we're eating more of the stuff that is making us sick. When we get clear on which foods are causing us challenges, we can return to that natural state of health in which we were designed to live. There is no greater investment we can make in living clean for life than identifying what not to eat by finding our toxic triggers.

## *Getting Clear on Your Toxic Triggers*

Not everyone has the same toxic triggers, but we do see patterns. Dr. Junger talked about the effects of gluten and dairy on the gut. Gluten and dairy are the two most common toxic triggers. But they aren't the only ones. In the previous chapter, Dr. Junger talked about corn, grains, soy, nightshades, alcohol, and processed sugar as potential toxic triggers. Foods affect everyone differently. These foods may or may not be toxic triggers for you, but you don't have to take our word for it. Living clean is all about figuring things out for yourself and seeing what works for you. The best method for being sure which foods are toxic triggers for you is by testing them. At the end of the Clean Gut program you went through the reintroduction process, which focused on gluten and dairy, the two most common toxic triggers. Having a good idea of how these two toxic triggers affect you means that you can see more clearly the connection between what you eat and how you feel.

## *Remove and Rotate*

Dr. Junger talked about this earlier, but it's worth revisiting. Once you understand how a specific food makes you feel, the next step is to practice removing and rotating that food. We say practice because rotating and removing toxic triggers is a process that won't happen overnight. A lot of the toxic triggers are addictive. They taste good, at least initially, and we're conditioned to seek them out when we're in search of comfort, a short-term high, or a treat. Be gentle with yourself during this process. Practice the remove and rotate steps listed in the reintroduction process to build new habits. Building new habits slowly, but with focused intention, will allow you to win in the long term.

Getting clear on what not to eat takes time and patience, but the return you'll get from your investment is incredible. So many of the health issues people deal with today are simply caused by the toxic triggers in their diet. Discovering your toxic triggers and taking steps to reduce their intake will radically alter your health for years to come. The goal here isn't to be a purist. The goal is to become clearer on the connection between what you eat and how you feel. With that knowledge, you are guaranteed to feel better, look better, and have the health you need to show up strong in every area of your life.

## What to Eat

Now that we've addressed what not to eat, we can explore what to eat. There are many different perspectives on what is the best diet for humans, but one thing every healthy dietary paradigm shares is the emphasis on whole foods; fresh, unprocessed foods are the foundation for long-term health. Let's be very clear on what we mean when we say whole foods. They are foods found in nature and made of one ingredient. Fruit, vegetables, meat, fish, dairy, eggs, grains, legumes, nuts, and seeds are the main foods that make up this category. As you can see, when we talk about whole foods, there are lots of foods to choose from.

Here's the caveat, though: eating a diet rich in whole foods is only a part of the bigger picture. Even if we eat lots of whole foods, it's important to eat whole foods minus our toxic triggers. This is where "what to eat" connects with "what not to eat." Find your toxic triggers, remove or rotate them in your diet, and eat whole, unprocessed, unrefined foods. If we don't remove our toxic triggers, we might still be eating certain whole foods that continue to throw off our health. A perfect example is gluten and dairy. They are both whole foods, but they are also highly allergenic foods. While this might sound confusing, it's really not. Think of it this way: the basic template for your long-term health is whole foods minus your toxic triggers.

At Clean, we have found that certain diets work best for certain people. Some people do better eating more animal protein; some do better eating less. Others find that a vegetarian or vegan diet is best for them. Each person has to discover what types of foods are best for him or her within the whole-foods category. This requires some experimentation and personal testing, which we'll address soon. But before we get into that, let's start with a step everyone can benefit from, no matter who you are: upgrading the quality of the whole foods you eat.

## Upgrade Your Whole Foods

Think of your body as the hardware of your computer. The food you eat is the software. This software gives your body information on how to run and which genetic switches to turn on or off. When you upgrade the quality of the food you eat, you in turn upgrade the quality of the information you send your body. As a result, your body runs better and becomes stronger.

Let's take a look at the ways you can upgrade your whole foods.

## FRUITS AND VEGETABLES

Purchase organic or chemical-free fruits and vegetables. Look for farmers' markets in your area. These fruits and vegetables are often free of pesticides and chemical treatments but are not labeled organic. Chat with your local farmer to find out how they grow their foods.

Try this: For the next month, when you buy your greens, buy only those labeled "organic" or buy them from a farmers' market. Over time, continue to increase the amount of organic whole foods in your diet.

## MEAT AND FISH

There are a lot of different ways to describe meat and fish. Look for the following labels to make sure you are getting the highest quality possible. The best meat you can purchase is organic, pasture-raised, and grass-fed. When it comes to fish, smaller cold-water fish are always a better option, because they are lower in heavy metals and toxins. Consider eating salmon, trout, mackerel, sardines, herring, and small halibut. Check out eatwild.com for a state-by-state listing of organic and grass-fed animal products.

Try this: If you typically eat meat at most meals, take one weekend to go vegetarian. Then try it for one week. Low energy, constipation, and bloating often occur at the extremes of dietary choices, so experimenting with adding or removing certain foods can teach you a lot about what your body needs. Stay open to the process and see what you learn.

## EGGS

Look for organic, free-range, and pasture-raised eggs. These eggs are more nutritious, higher in omega-3 fatty acids, and the hens' feed is free of genetically modified food. Pasture-raised eggs are the highest quality because the hens are raised on pastureland instead of in confinement, where they are fed primarily grains. The diet of pasture-raised hens is complemented with worms and bugs, which gives their eggs a higher nutrient profile for omega-3, vitamins A and E, and beta-carotene, an antioxidant and precursor to vitamin A production. Eggs from pasture-raised hens also have less cholesterol and saturated fat than conventional eggs.

Try this: In the next month, take a trip to your local farmers' market or health food store and look for pasture-raised eggs. They will be a dollar or two more expensive, but you'll provide your body with far more nutrition.

## GRAINS

If after the Clean Gut program you've reintroduced grains and found that they work for you, consider including nongluten grains in your diet, such as quinoa, millet, buckwheat, and rice. Soaking them overnight before cooking will make them easier to digest.

Try this: Once every month, for two to four days, go completely grain-free, both gluten (wheat, barley, rye) and nongluten (quinoa, rice, millet) varieties. Taking a break from consuming any grains is a great way to test whether grains are still working for you. Pay attention to changes in your skin, energy, digestion, and bowel movements.

## LEGUMES

Beans, lentils, and legumes are all useful sources of quality calories and protein. However they can be difficult for many people to digest. This is the reason we removed them from the Clean Gut program.

Try this: Next time you eat legumes, try soaking them first overnight. Notice if they are easier to digest.

## OILS

Look for organic expeller and cold-pressed, unrefined oils. Oils such as lard, coconut oil, and ghee are higher in saturated fats and are better for high-temperature cooking. Coconut oil is our recommendation as an all-purpose cooking oil and provides a good source of saturated fat. Olive oil is good for medium-temperature cooking but is best used in salad dressings or as a condiment. Nut and seed oils can provide fatty acids and nourishing fats but should not be used for cooking because they are unstable at high temperatures and will often turn rancid.

Try this: Use coconut oil for one week. Cook with it, use it as a skin moisturizer, and add it to shakes and recipes. Notice how you feel, the quality of your skin, and notice your digestion. Higher quality coconut oils will have less coconut taste. Check out cleangut.com for our favorite brands.

## NUTS AND SEEDS

Good sources of healthy fats and protein, nuts and seeds contain a wide range of vitamins and minerals. Look for raw varieties free of preservatives and sugar. Nuts and seeds can often be difficult to digest. Soaking them for a few hours can help. If you feel heavy after eating them, reduce the amount you include in your diet.

Try this: If you frequently rely on nuts and seeds as a daily snack, try reducing your quantity and frequency to one handful every other day. See if this improves your digestion.

• • •

Upgrading the quality of your food takes time; it's not something that can or needs to be done overnight. Keep making gradual changes each month until finally the food you eat is of the highest quality and can fully support your most important investment: your body and its ability to thrive.

## How to Eat

We've forgotten how to eat in a way that nourishes our bodies. Let's look at two reasons why that is.

First, junk and processed foods send the body mixed signals, causing us to overeat and become chemically addicted to these foods. Let's take processed sugar as an example. When the sweet receptors in the brain are overstimulated by sugar-rich foods, sugar easily overrides the mechanisms for self-control. After that first bite of ice cream or brownie, it's an uphill battle for most of us to stop.

The second reason is emotional. Since childhood, most of us have built emotional relationships to processed foods. Foods like ice cream and cake are used to celebrate important events or birthdays and to support us through difficult times. We've conditioned ourselves to reach for junk food, which causes a cascade of health issues. Processed foods are a part of holidays, funerals, vacations, and daily work breaks. We consume them when times are good, when times are bad, and when times are just plain boring. One of the most common times we eat emotionally is when a challenge presents itself. When a difficult event occurs—like a breakup or an argument—many of us reach for the classic "comfort foods," such as ice cream, which numb us from emotions we don't want to address. These comfort foods are so difficult to digest that they pull a good portion of the body's energy from its nervous system to its digestive system. A wave of sluggishness and calm comes over us; we no longer have the energy to think or feel the trigger issue that had caused the emotional response, and had prompted us to eat unhealthy food in the first place. Over time, we develop a habit of coping with emotions through unhealthy food, essentially forming a habit of emotional eating.

Poor quality, addictive foods and emotional eating have caused us to forget how to eat in a way that nourishes and supports our health. These two reasons have also made us forget how much and in what quantities to eat the whole foods that make up a healthy, long-term diet.

How much, then, should a person eat? How large or small a portion? How many times a day? And in what combinations? Diets have tried for years to determine in precise ways the exact amount and the exact way a person should eat each day. These types of plans often fail. This hyperattention to calories, nutrient levels, and weight loss creates a backlash: all the focus on portion sizes and body weight can easily diminish the pleasure we experience at each meal.

Let's look at five simple ideas that can help you sort through the noise, eat clean, and in the process find deep pleasure in a nourishing meal.

## 80-20

When your digestive system runs smoothly, you feel great and maintain a balanced energy level. When you overeat or eat foods in the wrong combinations, on the other hand, you put unneeded stress on your digestive tract. Overeating causes food to ferment, and this fermentation becomes food for yeast, fungus, and unwanted bacteria. As a result, you create an environment inside the gut that causes gas, bloating, constipation, and decreases absorption of nutrients from your food.

The 80-20 rule, as described in chapter 6, has two parts:

1. Fill 80 percent of your plate with greens and vegetables (raw, steamed, baked, cooked) and 20 percent with protein and good fats (meat, fish, quinoa, avocado, etc.).

2. Stop eating when you are 80 percent full. This is what the Japanese call *Hara Hachi Bu,* meaning "Eat until you are eight parts (out of ten) full." The long-living Okinawans, profiled in the book *The Blue Zones,* have used this technique for centuries to improve digestion and balance energy levels.

## Don't Food Bomb

Picture a typical holiday meal. Imagine a beautiful table full of a variety of breads, meats, cheeses, veggies, and wine. You eat a little bit of everything. Then dessert comes. You have some cake or cookies with ice cream topped off with some more alcohol and coffee. You feel a food coma setting in, and the indigestion and gas that often comes with it. The only thing you want to do is lie down and take a nap. This is what we call food bombing. A food bomb results from mixing too many different types of foods together in one meal. Each type of food requires different enzymes in order to be digested, so mixing too many together at once causes poor digestion and creates fatigue. This typical holiday meal might be an extreme example, but we go through some version of this every day. Let's take fruit, for example. Fruit takes the shortest time to digest and leaves the stomach within thirty minutes. When you eat fruit with protein or starches, the digestion of fruit can be held up and start to ferment in the intestines.

When fermentation happens in the gut, it reduces the assimilation of other nutrients at a meal and creates an environment that feeds yeast and fungus.

The same thing can occur when mixing animal protein with starches or grains. Meat, fish, and eggs require the secretion of hydrochloric acid and the enzyme pepsin. They break down the food in an acidic environment. Starches require the secretion of the enzyme ptyalin in an alkaline environment.

Mixing proteins and starches at the same meal can neutralize the breakdown of these foods and inhibit proper absorption, once again creating fermentation in the gut.

But a few simple guidelines will help you make food bombing a thing of the past and improve your digestion and health long term. When you combine food properly, you aid digestion and, most importantly, increase absorption of nutrients.

If you are tired of feeling bloated after every meal, it might be time to pay more attention to how you combine food. The best way to incorporate the following guidelines is to try them for a week. See how they affect your digestion and bowel movements. Once you get a taste of how great you can feel when your digestion runs optimally, you'll become addicted (in a good way) to eating foods that work well together.

Here are three simple guidelines to help eliminate your next food bomb:

1. Eat nonstarchy vegetables and leafy greens with animal protein, grains, rice, legumes, and starchy vegetables.

2. Avoid eating animal protein with grains, rice, or legumes.

3. Eat fruit alone.

Let's give a few examples:

| Foods | A Good Combination | Why? |
|---|---|---|
| Chicken and pasta | No | Animal proteins do not combine well with grains. |
| Fish and asparagus | Yes | Animal proteins combine well with veggies. |
| Quinoa and salad | Yes | Grains combine well with veggies. |

## A Shake a Day

A daily shake that includes good saturated fats and quality proteins is a simple way to keep your health on track. This habit is a quick and convenient way to start your morning. Rather than a traditional breakfast of energy-zapping muffins or bagels, a morning shake gives your body much-needed water, easily digestible nutrients, and sets the groundwork for clean eating habits throughout the rest of the day. Have a shake alone or as part of a clean breakfast. Use the shake recipes listed in the book (page 153) or discover new recipes at cleangut.com. Having this technique in your wellness toolbox will give you one more way to build a lifestyle that continues to increase your health year after year.

## Mastering Five Meals

Learning a new way of eating can be scary. If a food is unfamiliar to you, you may feel like you're being pushed outside your comfort zone. The idea of figuring out which foods to eat and how to prepare them can be overwhelming. The truth is that most people eat five to seven basic meals that they rotate seasonally. We may change the sauces, spices, and combinations, but the basic components of the meals are the same.

Instead of getting wrapped up in complex recipes or the fear of eating clean for the rest of your life, focus on mastering five healthy meals. These five meals will be the base of your diet, the food you'll eat most of the time. Discovering your five favorite meals will take some time, but once you do, you'll be able to use them as inspiration to create a lifetime of delicious and healthy meals.

## Personal Experimentation

The body is always changing and evolving. What works for you today may not work for you tomorrow. It's not a question of *if* this will happen to you; it is a question of *when* it will happen to you. At some point, foods you enjoyed often might start causing you issues. Or foods you never considered eating might help you evolve your health further.

The landscape of whole foods is a vast one with many different paths to take. In order to discover which whole foods to eat, how often, and how much, you will need to do some personal experimentation. Because everyone is different, what works for other people may not work for you. There are a variety of ways to experiment with the food you eat within the whole-foods-minus-toxic-triggers paradigm. Here are a few examples to get you started:

Try removing grains for two weeks.

Try removing corn and soy for two weeks.

Try adding a cup of fermented vegetables, kimchi, or sauerkraut each day to your dinner for a week.

Try adding one to two servings a day of a fresh green juice or green smoothie for two weeks.

When choosing a personal experiment, set a period of time to keep yourself focused. Then pay attention to your digestion, energy levels, bowel movements, mental clarity, and sense of well-being. If you are adding a new food to your diet frequently, notice what happens when you combine it with different foods. If you are removing a food, take notice of any emotional connections to the food or what feelings arise when it is gone.

With each personal experiment, you will gain greater awareness of your body and your needs, both physical and mental. The process is about paying attention to the close connection between what you eat and how you feel. The more you delve into this work, the more closely you build a lifestyle in line with who you really are and what you really want.

## Supplement Right

There is a lot of confusion about supplements. We have a simple philosophy at Clean: supplements help plug the nutritional gaps that keep us from reaching our health goals. While eating a clean, whole-foods diet is the most important first step, supplements can help correct nutritional deficiencies that have occurred as a result of poor lifestyle choices and impaired gut health. They can also make up for the nutrients and minerals much of our agricultural soil currently lacks. Overfarming, excessive application of pesticides and insecticides, and the use of genetically modified seeds often create more allergenic and less nutrient-dense foods. For example, magnesium is one of the major minerals lacking today in our soils and, as a result, it is one of the minerals people are most deficient in. When we replenish the nutrients through high-quality supplements, we can see our health improve. Like eating a clean diet, supplementation with key nutrients can support and build a sturdy foundation of health for years to come.

## Evolve and Change

Each person is different and so the best supplement programs will be tailored to your specific history and nutritional needs. One size does not fit all. For example, a person with chronic indigestion may have different needs from someone who does not. A heavy coffee drinker, with excessive stress and adrenal fatigue, will need different supplements from someone who has an autoimmune condition. Later in this section we outline the importance of getting tested, to figure out exactly what you need, but let's start with the supplements that can benefit most people right now. Remember, this is just a template, but in our experience, these are the supplements that will help the broadest number of people.

## Daily Supplements

These are the supplements we recommend most people take as a base for their wellness plan:

*Fish Oil (or Vegetarian Omega-3):* Both fish and algae varieties of omega-3 supplements provide essential fatty acids and reduce inflammation.

*Probiotics:* Beneficial bacteria help break down food, absorb nutrients, and boost immunity.

*Multivitamin-Multimineral:* A combination supplement replenishes essential vitamins and nutrients that may not be present in your diet.

*Vitamin D3:* This vitamin increases energy levels and immunity, boosts mood, and balances hormones. It can be found in capsule form or synthesized by your body during exposure to sunlight. When possible, focus on getting twenty minutes of sunlight on your bare skin.

*Magnesium:* An important mineral directly involved in over three hundred different bodily functions and often lacking in our diets.

For recommendations of our favorite brands and dosages, visit cleangut.com.

There is no fixed rule on how long to take these supplements. Many people continue to take them indefinitely. A good rule of thumb is to take them for three weeks, then take a few days off before starting them again.

## Gut-Specific Supplements

The following supplements will extend the efficacy of the Clean Gut program. They will build on the work you have already done and are specific to improving and maintaining gut health. The more you continue to support the health of the gut, the more your overall health will continue to benefit.

*Probiotics:* Stress, chlorinated water, polluted air, antibiotics, and chemicals in our food all present constant challenges to maintaining good bacteria. Increasing the amount of probiotics you take for a period of time can help deal with these challenges, improve digestion, and increase nutrient absorption.

*Prebiotics*: Prebiotics are sold as powders made from inulin and chicory root. They help promote the growth of bacteria in the digestive system and colon. Prebiotics are also found in raw Jerusalem artichoke, raw dandelion greens, raw garlic, raw leeks, and raw onions.

*Digestive Enzymes:* Digestive enzymes help your body digest fats, proteins, and carbohydrates. Take a digestive enzyme with meals to support optimum digestion.

*Hydrochloric Acid (HCL):* A critical component for proper digestion, HCL is useful for reducing upset stomach, nausea, and heaviness after eating.

*L-Glutamine:* This is an amino acid and the preferred food for intestinal cells. L-glutamine helps rebuild gut lining and restore gut integrity.

*Colostrum:* A form of milk produced by cows just before giving birth, colostrum has been shown to help restore gut health by repairing leaky gut. It contains growth factors, which heal damage to the intestinal lining, as well as large amounts of immunoglobulins, which help reduce harmful bacteria.

*Lactoferrin:* A glycoprotein derived from colostrum, lactoferrin has been shown to be antibacterial and supportive of the immune system. It also inhibits gut inflammation and has been used in the treatment and prevention of gastrointestinal inflammatory conditions.

*Fermented Foods:* These foods and drinks are easy to digest and contain beneficial bacteria and a wealth of B vitamins, minerals, and nutrients. When eating protein or fatty meals, add fermented foods to improve digestion. Look for raw, unpasteurized kimchi and sauerkraut, and low-sugar probiotic drinks. In addition, small amounts of kefir made from goat's milk or cow's milk may be useful, as long as dairy is not a trigger food for you.

## Get Tested

Tests help take the guesswork out of understanding how to improve our health. Today, we have incredible access to a number of tests that can help determine many obstacles or deficiencies in the body. It makes sense to utilize these tests whenever possible, because no one person has the same profile as the next. These tests are useful tools to help you maintain and improve upon the benefits of the Clean Gut program. Armed with clear information on a wide variety of data, you can catch imbalances early on, modify your diet and lifestyle, and create a personalized supplementation program that addresses your specific needs.

Here are three useful tests to begin with. Work with a functional medicine doctor in your area who is familiar with them and can order them for you (functionalmedicine.org).

*Gastrointestinal Profile Test:* This is a comprehensive stool analysis that will give a good snapshot of your gut health, including levels of bacteria, yeast, fungus, and parasites. It also shows absorption levels of fats and markers for inflammation. Our recommended test is Metametrix's GI Effects Complete Profile.

*Blood Panel:* Getting good blood work done is key. While most mainstream doctors order full blood panels, they are often not aware of the latest advances in testing. Working with a functional medicine doctor to get your blood work done will allow you to get a deeper understanding of your health.

*Heavy Metal Test:* This test looks for harmful levels of heavy metals, most notably lead and mercury. Mercury toxicity is called "the great mimicker" because it can show up as many different diseases, from psychiatric problems and cancers to autoimmune conditions. Take this test when your symptoms are not clear and do not seem to improve despite great efforts, or when you suspect exposure to heavy metals (via tuna or other mercury-laden fish, or silver amalgam dental fillings).

## Evaluating Your Test

The data you receive from your tests are only as useful as the healthcare practitioner who interprets them. Most mainstream doctors are not aware of the tests we just listed and do not know how to interpret them. For this reason, we recommend you seek out a functional medicine doctor in your area or a practitioner who is open to holistic practices. Using the tests we mentioned, your doctor will be better equipped to help you create a personalized plan that includes diet, supplements, stress management, and exercise.

•  •  •

Over time, your supplement routines will change. If you are healthy and exhibit few symptoms, the supplements we've described can be used as a starting place to help support your clean lifestyle. Unless you have created a plan with your functional medicine doctor, there is no set amount of time to use these supplements. Many people take them daily for years.

When testing a new supplement, a good rule of thumb is to take it alone with either water or food, depending on the directions, and take note of any reactions to it. If no duration of use is specified, try it for one to three months on a consistent basis and see if you notice any effects. Don't feel bad if you miss a day. Different holistic theories actually recommend taking breaks from supplements and taking them in different sequences—on for a few weeks, off for a week—in order to better absorb them.

Many of us on the Clean team have the habit of taking our supplements only during the week, not on the weekend. Once again, the main theme here is to use personal experimentation to find out what works best for you, while keeping in mind that what works for you today may not work for you tomorrow. Life and health are always developing, changing and transforming as you learn and grow. The more value you place on staying open and curious about your wellness path, the more you will develop flexible and robust health.

## Understand the Psychology of Clean Living

You may have heard the expression: 80 percent of what you do is psychology, 20 percent is taking action and following through. Regardless of the percentages, what this statement means is that a good part of what determines the vibrancy of your health is your thoughts about your health. Put another way, how you think about your health often determines your level of health.

One of the challenges to living clean is changing our habits. Habits take time to become ingrained, and during that period when we're learning how to do something new, there are ample opportunities to get off track. When we try to change a habit (e.g., eating better, removing a toxic trigger, exercising), we often bump up against ourselves. An event triggers something in us and we end up going back to the habits we are used to. While resistance to changing habits can happen in all areas of our lives (relationships, finances, career), for many of us food and emotional eating are the most challenging. Recognizing when and why we get off track and unpacking the emotional weight of these moments takes time.

Sometimes we don't know how to live healthier because there's an information gap. We are not sure what to do or how to follow through. But most of the time, we do know what works; we just have trouble making the necessary changes. The yo-yoing back and forth between following a wellness program and not following it creates something we call the cycle of emotional eating. When we enter this cycle, poor habits create more poor habits, and we cycle downward. It's like compound debt. If we miss a few payments on a credit card, we begin to pay penalties on what we owe. And then we pay penalties on the penalties. This vicious cycle causes immense amounts of stress and requires huge amounts of energy to break it.

If you understand the cycle of emotional eating—why it happens, how it works, and what you can do when you recognize it in your life—you turn the cycle that spirals downward on its head, sending the spiral upwards. The opposite of compound debt is compound interest. When you earn interest on money, that interest compounds and begins to make money on itself. Interest starts making more interest. If you are aware of the cycle of emotional eating, then you can interrupt it before it wreaks havoc, and like compound interest, your healthy habits will encourage new healthy habits with less energy and less need for willpower alone.

## The Cycle of Emotional Eating

There are four main phases of emotional eating: the trigger, the cover up, the false bliss, and the hangover.

> *Trigger:* A "trigger" is an event or situation that causes a stressful or painful emotional response. Caroline was trying to change her habit of eating junk food whenever she felt sad. We worked with her to get clear on what her specific trigger was. We asked her to describe specifically what happened before she began to emotionally overeat. She told us once that her boyfriend had canceled a special date they had been planning for some time. Her trigger

event was her boyfriend's cancellation, but it was her pain and emotional response to that trigger that started a cycle of emotional eating. We asked her what she felt when he canceled. She said, "I felt sad, and then I felt like I wasn't enough for him." Caroline found these feelings painful to experience. Instead of giving herself space to truly feel what she was feeling, she unconsciously committed to avoiding the pain and seeking momentary pleasure to suppress the feelings. We call this the "cover up."

Before we describe the cover up, however, let's take a closer look at a few more elements of the trigger, so you can recognize it when it shows up. Recognizing a trigger will help you interrupt a cycle before it starts. Any object, any event, any conversation can be made into a trigger. Triggers create a physical response in the body. Your breathing may speed up or become shallow; you may start sweating. Emotionally, you might feel angry, sad, or annoyed. Why you have certain triggers as opposed to others has to do with your family history, your personality, and your insecurities. Working with a coach or therapist can help you uncover why a trigger exists or is so pronounced, but for now, let's begin with the recognition of your triggers when they occur.

*Cover Up:* Because Caroline did not give herself permission to feel her "I'm not enough" feelings, she unconsciously covered them up with food. There are many ways to cover up feelings you don't want to feel, but one of the most common ways is to eat foods high in sugar, high in carbohydrates, and high in fat, such as ice cream, cakes, and cookies. These classic comfort foods are aptly named because they hide the difficult feelings by producing a momentary sense of calm. When you eat difficult-to-digest and highly allergenic foods, two important things happen. First, the allergenic part of gluten, dairy, and sugar creates an adrenaline effect. This adrenaline immediately makes you feel better. This is one of the primary reasons that the most common toxic triggers are hard to reduce or remove from your diet. They make you feel great at first but leave you feeling terrible later. Second, classic comfort foods are heavy and difficult to digest. Apart from the brain, digestion demands as much energy as it can get. Heavy foods pull energy from your nervous system, where you feel your feelings, and direct it toward digestion. These foods cover up emotions, creating a numbing effect for the feelings that started the cycle in the first place.

*False Bliss:* After the habitual and unconscious decision is made to eat in order to cover up your feelings, you enter the "false bliss" stage. In Caroline's example, when she eats ice cream and processed chocolate, she numbs her painful feelings and then experiences a high from the sugar-rich, dairy-rich foods. Characteristics of this stage are a sensation that everything is fine, that there was no issue to deal with in the first place, or that it was just a figment of your imagination. The comfort food paired with the desire to cover up enables you to forget, at least for a short while.

*Hangover:* Soon, the sensation of bliss and forgetting starts to wear off and the "hangover" sets in. An hour later, Caroline begins to feel sick in her stomach. She feels bloated, gassy, and tired. She wonders why she went this far, again, why she got off track when she was feeling so good and eating clean. She feels guilt and shame. Two types of pain occur during the hangover. There is the physical pain and discomfort, which occurs after eating too much of a toxic trigger or poor combinations of foods. Then there is the emotional pain, which comes from feeling guilt and shame about not doing what you had originally set out to do (eat clean), repeating a well-worn pattern. On top of all that, you can often feel confused, because you have forgotten the original trigger that started the downward cycle in the first place.

## The Cycle Continues

Caroline's guilt and shame caused her to turn this incident into a new trigger. She felt bad about not continuing with her wellness plan and, because this had happened before, it reinforced her belief that she would never get healthy and that eating clean was just too hard. These feelings caused her to enter a downward spiral during the next few days. She repeatedly ate poorly, even though she knew it was not helping. She just couldn't seem to stop. Finally, a few weeks later she called us to help her get back on track. Her thought was that she just lacked discipline. The truth was that she was caught in a cycle of emotional eating. Now it was time to break the cycle.

## Breaking the Cycle

Breaking free from the cycle of emotional eating begins with understanding the pattern and committing yourself to recognizing it when it shows up. By becoming aware of the cycle and reflecting on specific moments when you have been caught in it, you can begin to catch yourself earlier and earlier. Now that you know the names of the different phases, you can identify them when they show up in your life, and call them out in your mind, *Oh yes, here it is again. I am covering it up!* Over time, these patterns no longer sneak up on you. Once you recognize how these patterns have occurred in your life, how they have pulled you away from where you want to go and who you really want to become, their seductive power loses its pull.

Awareness is the first and most important step. With attention, you will learn more about the ways you personally use this cycle and the stories and tricks you tell yourself to justify not committing to your potential. The awareness you develop over time will aid you in using the following three additional ways to break the cycle.

### ADDRESS THE ISSUE DIRECTLY

The simplest and most direct way to interrupt the cycle is to address the issue directly when you feel triggered. If the trigger was an offhanded comment by a coworker, you might ask to speak to that coworker about it, even though a part of you feels scared to talk to them. Often emotional-eating cycles can be stopped in their tracks when the initial triggers are addressed honestly. If you are unable to speak directly to a person, or the trigger is an object, like an old picture of a relative or the memories of a partner, take a moment to fully feel what you are feeling. The awareness that you are being triggered, plus the permission to fully feel what you feel, will lessen the power of the cycle of emotional eating.

Brad Blanton's *Radical Honesty* and Susan Campbell's *Getting Real* are two wonderful books to help you with the process of honest communication.

### BUILD A TOOLBOX OF HEALTHY HABITS

Once you are aware of your triggers, you'll notice your old habits trying to pull you in a familiar direction. You will notice yourself craving foods that you have built up an emotional relationship with in the past. Transitioning from these foods and old habits is a process. Often when you first notice a trigger, you don't have healthy new practices ready to put into action. Even when you are clear about that trigger, without a means to redirect your energy you may unknowingly fall back into the old habit.

A toolbox of healthy habits works best when you enjoy them, but remember that in the initial phases your old habits will do their best to make you think the new habits are boring and unpleasant. Don't let this stop you. Take a leap of faith and commit to using these tools when you feel triggered. If you fall back into the cycle, use them the next time. Keep using them until they become a reflex, so when you feel triggered you instantly know what to do.

Once you have utilized these new habits, your old habits— the one's that kept you from growing—will fade naturally into the background. Soon, you will only hear the faint rumblings of who you once were, and you'll be in a stronger place to continue to make forward progress on your health.

Here are a few of our favorite healthy habits. These habits will nourish you and encourage you to stay on track:

Take a walk.

Drink water or a green juice.

Take a nap.

Do something nice for someone.

Have a clean snack.

### GET TO THE ROOT

At the base of our emotions and habits are events in our past and stories about those events that we have internalized. These internalized stories create the program that runs many of our most common habits. When certain habits are not working for us, when they cause us pain and keep us from progressing toward our goals, time needs to be taken to try to understand and reflect on them. Getting to the root means asking ourselves some deep questions about why we do the things we do. And more often than not, the reason we try to numb our feelings with food is due to fear or insecurity.

In Caroline's example, the fact that she reached for junk food when her boyfriend canceled their plans is rooted in her fear of being alone. When she asked herself why being alone produced such intense fear, she recognized that she feared not being able to take care of herself. Once she recognized these feelings and allowed herself to feel the fear she had tried to cover up, the fear began to lessen. As she became clearer about the root of her emotional eating, she became better at interrupting the cycle before it started and substituting new healthy habits for her junk-food eating.

Getting to the root of our emotional relationships to food and the ways in which we use the cycle of emotional eating to hide our feelings is a lifelong project. Personal reflection, supported by coaches, therapists, and holistic health practitioners, is a real and useful way to grow beyond common triggers. The more we give this work attention, patiently and compassionately, the more we reset how we live to be more in line with the way we really want to live. For most people, this means more joy, more energy, more awareness, and ultimately better health. And all of this work—the building of awareness, the untangling of our complex relationships to our habits, and the substituting of new habits for old ones—leads us to do what we are most excited about at Clean: take care of our health so we can live well, live strong, and live better.

# Move and Chill

Exercise and rest are two of the most fundamental practices for living clean for life. They also cost the least and can help us make serious gains in our health, if we give them some attention. This is easy in theory: find one of the hundreds of exercise programs out there and do it, get enough sleep each night, and reduce the amount of stress in your life. We've all heard this advice time and time again. But the truth is we often don't act on it. So let's try telling a different story.

We evolved in a very different environment from the environment we live in today. We evolved in a world where we moved a lot, rarely had access to continuous food supplies, and were relatively free of chronic stress. But for most of us in developed countries, we now live in a world that our Paleolithic ancestors could hardly imagine—a world where food is always accessible, where a lot of movement is not necessary to get the basic necessities of life, and where chronic stress is the norm. In essence, we have created a world our genes have always wanted, an environment where we save our energy for dangerous situations (which rarely occur anymore, but our genes don't know that), where food is abundantly available, and where we can access media and means of communication however and whenever we want. So, it makes sense why we may have difficulty getting ourselves to move more, refrain from overeating junk food, and unplug ourselves from our toys. It's not what our genes want. As far as our genetic impulses are concerned, we've basically run across the finish line and are stuffing our faces full of never-ending cake.

But the question remains: Now what? If we have crossed the finish line, and there is nothing left for us to do, then that's it. Game over. The increasing incidents of chronic disease confirm this, and they also confirm that we have some work to do. The next step is for us to get back in the race. That means, getting back to moving more and resting more. We are meant to both move and chill. It's part of our genetic history to get moving and then balance the movement with periods of deep relaxation and lots of sleep. Think of moving and chilling as food, part of your daily nourishment, free for the taking whenever you want them.

The good thing about getting back into the race is that most of the time it actually feels good. When we exercise, we burn fat and excess weight, create endorphins, which make us feel great and improve our mood, and build strength and endurance. When we get enough sleep, and unplug, we give ourselves time to recharge and reflect. Both moving and chilling directly help us reduce the amount of stress in our lives and make us better at handling stress when it does occur.

The major challenge with getting back in the race is that we often try to take on too much at once. When we take on unrealistic goals, such as losing twenty pounds or completely transforming our bodies in a week, we set ourselves up for failure. And with failure comes guilt and shame, hardly a good motivator to continue with a program. Small habits done consistently tend to work best. Focus on the "minimum viable dose," the smallest amount needed to get you started, and then stick with that for twenty-one days. For example, a consistent walk after dinner each night or one minute of focus on your breath can build the lasting foundation for an entire exercise or meditation program. The key idea is that something small when done consistently produces big results down the line.

Each time you practice a small habit (e.g., meditation, walk, or exercise routine), congratulate yourself. Give yourself a physical pat on the back to celebrate. It's a small act, but that's the point—the more you take pleasure in your small habit, the more it will stick with you. Then add other habits or increase the amount of time you do them. A simple walk can turn into a running program or a day hike. A minute of meditation can turn into a consistent place of respite you can go to reduce stress and fatigue in your life.

Whatever method of exercise or stress reduction you choose, know that it is not only an integral part of living clean for life but also an integral part of who you are. Moving and chilling are genetic impulses that are ready for the taking whenever you are. They are only asking for one thing: start small and start now.

## Create Community

Communities are a place for like-minded people to share their ideas and grow from the perspective of others. No matter how smart you are or how many books you have on your bookshelf, there's nothing like being part of a group of people who value what you value and can offer you advice when you are stuck, especially when it comes to your wellness journey.

All too often people try to get and stay healthy on their own, without the support of others. When swimsuit season nears and your motivation is high, you might be focused. But what happens when your motivation shifts, or life gets tough, or you can hide beneath layers and layers of clothing? Being part of a wellness community can provide support when you need it most.

When we interviewed members of our Clean community for this book, we found that the people who reported feeling the happiest about their health were part of strong communities. Online communities are especially great, because regardless of where you live you can connect and learn from people from all over the world. Our own Clean community has more than fifty thousand people in it from more than a hundred different countries. Being part of a thriving online community can make it easier to connect with people in your area too. Many members of our community have told us that they've met and connected with others in their area, who they first met online.

People who budget, save their money, and then go on to become very wealthy are often friends with other people who are also wise with their money. People who are big spenders, never save, and continuously mismanage their money usually hang out with others who do the same. Our community shapes us and makes us either better or worse. Truly healthy people have healthy friends who like discussing what they do to stay healthy—not in an obsessive way, but in a fun way, which reinforces continuous growth and focus.

No matter how inspired or disciplined you are about your diet or wellness program, at some point you'll get off track. This is natural and, in fact, it happens to everyone, including authors of health books. Yet very few people talk about this openly or about how to address it. We feel community is a major part of the solution.

Getting off track isn't a bad thing. We often make it a bad thing with our feelings of shame, guilt, and blame, but the truth is a lot of lessons can be learned when it happens. Learning those lessons on your own can be tough. Being part of a community helps you put those lessons into perspective and allows you to come up with real solutions to try, which have worked for others.

# Final Thoughts

The guiding principles for living clean for life are clear and direct concepts that have worked for our community and our team. That being said, there is no single right or optimal way for everyone. There are hundreds of programs, doctors, and "experts" who tell us what to eat and how to live. But nothing is more powerful than your personal experience as you test and try out each of these principles. Pick the ones that work for you and modify the ones that don't. Most importantly, though, if something isn't working for you, be open and willing to try something new.

# Clean Gut Recipes

Welcome to the Clean Kitchen! The following recipes have been created specifically for the Clean Gut program by the resident Clean Chefs. We spent lots of time creating these recipes to be easily digested and low-glycemic. We're happy to share them and help make the food piece of this program as easy and enjoyable as possible.

With a variety of vegetables, grass-fed, free-range meats, eggs, nuts, and seeds, the Clean Gut program is not only healing and nourishing but tasty.

We hope you take these recipes, experiment, and make them your own, using the foods that are local and seasonal where you live.

Have fun, get creative, and if you need more inspiration, you can sign up for a new recipe every week delivered directly to your inbox at cleangut.com.

—Chef Jenny Nelson and Chef Shannon Sinkin

# RECIPE GUIDELINES

*Nuts:* use raw or dry-roasted, unsalted

*Nut or seed butter:* use unsweetened, unsalted, raw or dry-roasted, organic when possible

*Non-dairy milks:* use unsweetened and free of xanthum gum

*Protein powder:* rice, hemp, or pea based protein, no soy

*Coconut flakes:* unsweetened

*Coconut water and coconut milk:* unsweetened, no added flavor, organic when possible

*Berries:* fresh or frozen, no added sweetener

*Chicken, duck, and turkey:* free-range or organic

*Fish:* cold-water, wild caught

*Beef and lamb:* grass-fed

*Eggs:* cage-free, organic

*Broth or stock:* free-range or organic, use homemade if possible, see our recipes for beef broth and chicken stock

# SHAKES

During the 21-Day Clean Gut program you'll have a shake for breakfast. These shake recipes, which are full-on meal replacements, have been designed to be nutrient rich and delicious.

When it comes to ingredients, feel free to switch the ingredients listed in the recipes for what you have on hand. For example, if you can't find coconut milk, simply use almond milk. Or if you don't enjoy almond butter than you can use cashew butter instead. If you have a nut allergy, use sunflower seed butter or coconut manna. Many of our recipes use nuts, but it's very possible to do the cleanse without using them. Simply omit from the recipe or substitute with a similar product.

## Basic Nut Milk
(Makes 4 cups)

This recipe makes the almond milk used in some of the following recipes. Use any type of nut or seed except peanuts.

> 1 cup nuts, soaked for 3 hours in purified water, then drained
> 1 teaspoon vanilla extract
> Stevia to taste
> 3 cups purified water

1. In a blender, purée all the ingredients for about 3 minutes.

2. Strain the mixture through a fine-mesh strainer or cheesecloth.

3. Store in the refrigerator. The milk will keep for three to four days.

## Becky's Morning Shake
(Serves 1 to 2)

> 8 ounces purified water
> 3 to 4 ounces non-dairy milk
> 2 loosely packed cups spinach
> Flesh of ½ avocado
> 2 tablespoons almond butter
> 1 tablespoon protein powder
> 2 teaspoons ground flax seed or meal
> Pinch of sea salt
> Stevia to taste
> Optional: 1 tablespoon carob powder or raw cacao powder

In a blender, purée all the ingredients until smooth and creamy.

## Green Coco Shake
(Serves 1)

> 2 cups coconut water
> Flesh of 1 ripe avocado
> 1 tightly packed cup of fresh spinach
> 3 heaping tablespoons cashews
> Stevia to taste

In a blender, purée all the ingredients until smooth and creamy.

## Creamy Blueberry Shake
(Serves 1)

> 1½ cups coconut milk
> ½ cup fresh or frozen blueberries
> ¼ cup organic almond butter
> 1 tablespoon chia seed gel*
> 2 loosely packed cups dark leafy greens (spinach, kale, etc.)
> Stevia to taste

In a blender, purée all the ingredients until smooth and creamy, roughly 45 seconds.

*To make the chia seed gel, soak ¼ cup chia seeds in 1 cup purified water for at least 30 minutes to 1 hour. Chia absorbs a lot of water, so if the gel becomes too thick simply add more water. Soaked chia is easier to digest and blends more smoothly than unsoaked chia. The gel will keep for a week in the fridge.

## Chocolate Mint Nut Shake
(Serves 1)

> 1 cup coconut milk
> 1 tablespoon vanilla extract
> 2 tablespoons raw cacao powder or carob powder
> 2 to 4 tablespoons nut butter (a handful of raw or roasted nuts will work also)
> 1 to 2 tablespoons liquid mint-flavored chlorophyll
> Stevia to taste
> Optional: 1 to 2 tablespoons plant-based protein powder
> Optional: 1 tablespoon ground flax seeds or meal

In a blender, purée all the ingredients until smooth and creamy.

## Chocolate-Covered Blueberry Shake
(Serves 1 to 2)

> 1 large handful frozen blueberries
> 1 to 2 tightly packed cups fresh spinach
> 2 tablespoons almond butter
> 1 tablespoon raw cacao powder or carob powder
> Dash of ground cinnamon, to taste
> 1 cup coconut milk
> 1 cup coconut water, or purified water*
> Stevia to taste
> Optional: 1 to 2 tablespoons plant-based protein powder
> Optional: 1 tablespoon ground flax seeds or meal

In a blender, purée all the ingredients until smooth and creamy.

*You could replace the coconut water with an herbal or green tea.

## Vanilla Almond Shake
(Serves 1)

> 2 cups almond milk
> 1 tablespoon vanilla extract
> 1 heaping tablespoon almond butter
> 1 teaspoon ground cinnamon
> ½ teaspoon ground nutmeg
> 1 teaspoon spirulina powder
> Dash of sea salt
> Optional: stevia to taste

In a blender, purée all the ingredients until smooth and creamy.

## Chocolate Ginger Shake
(Serves 1)

 1 cup unsweetened chocolate almond milk
 1-inch fresh ginger piece, peeled and finely minced,
   saving any juice that comes from it, or 1 tablespoon
   ginger powder
 ½ teaspoon ground cardamom
 1 heaping tablespoon raw cacao powder or cocoa powder
 1 heaping tablespoon almond or cashew butter
   (unsweetened sunflower seed butter will work too)
 1 to 2 teaspoons liquid chlorophyll or spirulina powder
 Stevia to taste

In a blender, purée all the ingredients until smooth and creamy.

# SOUPS

## Zucchini Mushroom Soup
(Serves 2 to 4)

> 2 tablespoons coconut oil
> 6 cups chopped mushrooms, such as crimini or portobello
> 1 red or yellow onion, roughly chopped
> 2 garlic cloves, chopped or crushed
> 1 large zucchini, cut into ½-inch-thick rounds
> 1 bay leaf
> Water as needed
> 2 cups chopped cauliflower
> Optional: approximately 1 cup almond milk, or an additional 2 tablespoons coconut oil (for thicker consistency)
> Sea salt to taste
> Freshly ground black pepper to taste
> Chopped fresh rosemary, sage, thyme, or parsley for garnish (optional, but recommended)

1. In a large soup pot set over medium-high heat, melt the coconut oil. Stir in the mushrooms and a sprinkle of sea salt. Sauté until the mushrooms are lightly brown, about 3 to 4 minutes.

2. Stir in the onion, garlic, and zucchini, and cook an additional 3 to 4 minutes.

3. Add the bay leaf and enough water to just cover the vegetables. Cover the pot and bring to a gentle boil. Then lower the heat to medium-low and cook for an additional 12 minutes.

4. Add the cauliflower and continue to cook until the cauliflower is soft. Remove the pot from the heat.

5. Purée the soup with an immersion blender, or in batches in a high-speed blender, until the mixture is creamy. For

a richer taste, add the optional almond milk or optional coconut oil.

6. Return the soup to the pot and season to taste with salt and pepper.

7. Serve warm, garnished with the fresh herbs of your choice.

## Spinach Avocado Soup
(Serves 2 to 4)

2 cups unsweetened coconut milk*
Juice of 1 lime or lemon
2 ripe avocados, cut into large chunks
2 handfuls fresh baby spinach
¼ cup fresh cilantro leaves
1 garlic clove
2 tablespoons minced shallot
Sea salt to taste

1. In a blender, purée all the ingredients until smooth and creamy.

2. Garnish with additional cilantro leaves or chopped avocado, or with nuts or seeds of your choice and serve chilled or at room temperature.

*To make fresh coconut milk, in a blender purée 1 cup shredded unsweetened coconut with 2 cups water for 45 seconds. Strain the mixture through a fine-mesh strainer or cheesecloth.

You can use canned coconut milk, but it's very rich and some brands may have additives. Read the ingredients and, when in doubt, make your own. You can also use coconut milk in a carton from the health-food or grocery store. Make sure it's unsweetened. Coconut milk will store for several days in the fridge.

## Cucumber Dill Bisque with Hard-Boiled Eggs
(Serves 2 as a meal or 4 as a side or starter)

    3 tablespoons extra-virgin olive oil
    2 small cucumbers, peeled and roughly chopped
    1 cup chicken or vegetable broth
    1 tablespoon chopped fresh dill, or 2 teaspoons dried
    ½ cup coconut milk (the thicker kind from a can)
    Sea salt and freshly ground black pepper to taste
    4 eggs, hard-boiled and peeled

1. Heat the olive oil in a medium saucepan, add the cucumber, and simmer for a few minutes, until the cucumber pieces start to soften just a bit.

2. Add the broth and continue to simmer for an additional 12 minutes.

3. Stir in the dill and the coconut milk. Once the coconut milk is warm, salt and pepper the soup to taste.

4. Slice each hard-boiled egg in half and put two halves each in the bottoms of four serving bowls.

5. Ladle the soup over each set of halves and garnish with extra dill and cracked pepper.

6. Serve warm, but you can also serve this chilled in the warmer months.

# Thai Coconut Chicken Soup
(Serves 2 to 4)

2 to 3 tablespoons coconut oil

2 garlic cloves, minced

½ red onion, chopped

1 jalapeño pepper, seeded and minced (use less if you are sensitive to spice)

16 ounces coconut milk (can or carton)

4 cups vegetable or chicken broth

2-inch fresh ginger piece, peeled and grated

2 lemongrass stalks, cut into chunks and bruised with the back of a knife to bring out the flavor

Juice and zest of 1 lime

3 to 4 tablespoons fish sauce (Red Boat brand), starting with 3 tablespoons, adding more to taste

1 pound boneless chicken breast, sliced thinly

1 cup chopped mushrooms, any variety

8 cherry tomatoes, halved

Dash of stevia (to taste; start with a tiny amount, as it's very sweet)

Chopped fresh cilantro leaves, for garnish

Wheat-free tamari to taste

1. In a soup pot, melt the coconut oil.

2. Add the garlic, onion, and jalapeño, and sauté until the mixture is fragrant, about 2 minutes.

3. Then add the coconut milk, broth, ginger, lemongrass, lime zest (reserving the juice for later), fish sauce, and chicken.

4. Simmer 15 minutes.

5. Then add the lime juice, mushrooms, tomatoes, and stevia, and simmer an additional 5 minutes.

6. Serve garnished with cilantro and add a splash of wheat-free tamari, if additional salt is desired.

## Creamy Roasted Tomato Soup
(Serves 2 to 4)

  8 medium tomatoes (any kind), roughly chopped
  3 to 4 garlic cloves, minced
  1 yellow onion, roughly chopped into large chunks
  3 teaspoons fresh thyme
  3 tablespoons extra-virgin olive oil
  Sea salt and freshly ground black pepper to taste
  3 cups vegetable broth
  1 cup coconut milk
  Optional: ½ teaspoon red pepper flakes
  Optional: 10 to 12 leaves fresh basil, chopped for garnish

1. Preheat the oven to 400°F.

2. In a roasting pan, toss together the tomatoes, garlic, onion, thyme, and olive oil, and salt and pepper the mixture to taste.

3. Bake in the oven until the tomatoes, garlic, and onion start to caramelize, probably about 50 minutes, stirring occasionally to prevent burning.

4. Transfer all the contents of the pan to a soup pot, including the roasting juices.

5. Stir in the broth, cover, and bring the pot to a boil.

6. Then reduce the heat to low and simmer 30 minutes.

7. Remove the pot from the heat. Using either an immersion blender or a traditional blender, processing the soup in batches once it has cooled enough to handle, purée the soup until it's smooth.

8. Stir in the coconut milk and optional red pepper flakes, if desired.

9. Reheat it in the pot before serving garnished with the basil.

# Curried Fish Chowder

(Serves 2 to 4)

   2 small parsnips, peeled and roughly chopped
   3 tablespoons extra-virgin olive oil
   1 yellow onion, roughly chopped
   3 garlic cloves, minced
   1 fennel bulb, thinly sliced
   2 leeks, the white parts thinly sliced into rounds, the
      green parts discarded
   2 celery stalks, cut into small chunks
   2 cups water
   8 ounces chicken or vegetable broth
   1 heaping tablespoon curry powder
   1 pound boneless white fish, such as haddock, cod, or
      halibut, cut into chunks
   2 cups coconut milk
   4 ounces anchovies, water or oil packed, or fresh
   ½ teaspoon sea salt, or to taste
   ½ teaspoon freshly ground black pepper to taste

1. In a medium pot, cover the parsnips with several inches
   of water, bring to a boil, and cook until the parsnips
   are tender. Then remove the pot from heat, drain the
   parsnips, and set aside.

2. Meanwhile, in a large soup pot, heat the olive oil and
   sauté the onion, garlic, fennel, leeks, and celery over
   medium heat, stirring frequently until the vegetables are
   tender and the onions have begun to brown.

3. Add the 2 cups water, broth, and curry powder.

4. Bring to a boil, then reduce the heat, cover, and simmer 8
   to 10 minutes, until the vegetables are thoroughly cooked.

5. Add the fish chunks. When the pieces turn opaque, add
   the coconut milk, anchovies, and the cooked parsnips.

6. Simmer approximately 6 to 8 minutes until everything is
   warm and fully cooked.

7. Season with the salt and pepper, and serve warm. If you like, garnish each bowl with a drizzle of olive oil and an extra dash of curry powder.

## Pumpkin Curry Soup
(Serves 2 to 4)

2 cups peeled and diced butternut squash
2 to 4 tablespoons extra-virgin olive oil, plus extra for the roasting
Sea salt
1 yellow onion, roughly chopped
3 garlic cloves, minced
2 tablespoons minced fresh ginger
1 15- or 16-ounce can pumpkin purée
2 cups vegetable or chicken broth
1 cup coconut milk
1 heaping tablespoon curry powder
Pinch of cayenne
Juice of 1 lime, or to taste
Optional: chopped scallions or fresh cilantro leaves for garnish

1. Preheat the oven to 450°F.

2. In a roasting pan, toss the butternut chunks with a splash of olive oil and salt to taste.

3. Roast until the squash pieces are tender and dark brown, about 30 minutes. Set aside.

4. Meanwhile, in a soup pot heat the olive oil over medium-low heat.

5. Sauté the onion and garlic, stirring frequently, for 8 to 10 minutes.

6. Add the ginger and continue sautéing and stirring until everything is tender and turning golden. You don't want the garlic and ginger to get too dark and crispy, though, so keep the heat low and watch as you stir.

7. Then stir in the pumpkin purée, broth, coconut milk, curry powder, and cayenne. Stir a few times, then let the mixture simmer on low heat an additional 20 minutes.

8. Add the roasted squash and a few splashes of lime juice, or to taste.

9. When everything is warm and cooked thoroughly, serve in bowls.

10. Garnish with scallions or cilantro, if you wish.

# FISH ENTRÉES

## Hemp Pesto–Smothered Halibut
(Serves 4)

½ cup hemp seeds
1 garlic clove, diced
Juice of 1 medium lemon
½ cup fresh basil leaves
1 to 2 teaspoons sea salt
Freshly ground black pepper to taste
¼ cup extra-virgin olive oil, plus extra to dress the fish
1 pound halibut, or any wild-caught cold-water fish, cut into 4 fillets
2 lemons, thinly sliced
2 large handfuls lettuce greens, dressed with fresh lemon juice

1. Preheat the oven to 350°F.

2. First, make the pesto. Place the hemp seeds, garlic, and basil in a food processor and pulse until finely chopped.

3. Add the lemon juice, salt, and pepper. Keep processing while drizzling in the olive oil. For this dish, the pesto is best on the thicker side, so only add enough oil to purée the mixture well.

4. Set aside.

5. Coat the fish fillets with some olive oil, and salt and pepper to taste. Cover each with thin slices of lemon.

6. Place the fillets in a baking dish lined with parchment paper, or lightly oiled, and bake 10 to 25 minutes, or until the fish is cooked through (check with a fork).

7. Divide the lettuce greens between four servings plates, dressing with fresh lemon juice if you wish.

8. Top each with a halibut fillet.

9. Place a scoop of pesto on each fillet, and spread to coat the fillet.

10. Serve warm.

## Spicy Herb Poached Fish
(Serves 2)

½ bunch fresh cilantro
½ bunch fresh Italian parsley
10 garlic cloves
1 lemon, sliced
3 serrano peppers, seeded and roughly chopped
½ pound halibut or other steak-like fish (salmon works too)
1 teaspoon sea salt
½ teaspoon freshly ground black pepper

*Cooking Liquid*
1 cup extra-virgin olive oil
1 cup water
1 teaspoon sea salt
¼ teaspoon freshly ground black pepper
½ teaspoon paprika
Optional: ½ teaspoon cayenne

1. Lay the sprigs of cilantro and parsley in the bottom of a pot with a lid.

2. Scatter the garlic cloves, lemon slices, and chopped peppers on them.

3. Season the fish with the salt and pepper and place it on top in a single layer. Set the pan aside.

4. To make the cooking liquid, in a small bowl whisk together the olive oil, water, salt, pepper, paprika, and optional cayenne.

5. Pour the liquid over the fish.

6. Bring the pot to a boil, then cover and reduce the heat.

7. Simmer 5 minutes, then remove the lid and increase the heat to medium-high.

8. Cook the fish until the cooking liquid reduces, about 15 minutes.

9. Serve warm with any remaining sauce spooned over the fish.

## Rice-Free Salmon Sushi
(Serves 2)

½ pound wild-caught salmon fillet (canned salmon will work too, but fresh is better)

1 scallion, chopped

1 small avocado, mashed

Optional: ½ sheet nori paper, crumbled (optional, but recommended!)

Wheat-free tamari to taste

1 English cucumber, sliced into 1-inch-thick rounds (you can peel if you want, or leave unpeeled)

Optional: pickled ginger, unsweetened*

1. In a frying pan, poach the salmon in 1 inch of water until just cooked, about 2 minutes on each side, depending on the thickness. (Or you may grill it, if you prefer, for the same amount of time.)

2. Remove the bones and flake the salmon apart.

3. In a bowl, mash together the salmon, scallion, avocado, nori, and tamari until blended.

4. Hollow out the seeded area of each slice of cucumber with a sharp knife, creating rings.

5. Fill each ring with the salmon mixture.

6. Serve with pickled ginger and extra tamari, if desired.

*Look for brands without preservatives, dyes, or MSG.

## Lemon Dijon Haddock
(Serves 2 to 4)

> 1 pound haddock fillet (cod or any other mild white cold-water fish will work too)
> 1 to 2 tablespoons Dijon mustard
> 2 tablespoons coconut oil, melted, plus extra for greasing the pan
> 1 cup almond flour
> 1 small handful minced fresh parsley leaves
> Juice and zest of 1 lemon
> Sea salt to taste

1. Preheat the oven to 350°F.

2. Oil a baking dish with olive oil or coconut oil.

3. Place the fish in a single layer in the dish.

4. Spread a thin layer of mustard on top of the fish, and set aside.

5. In a small bowl, combine the melted coconut oil, almond flour, parsley, lemon juice and zest, and salt the mixture to taste.

6. Coat the fish with the crumb mixture.

7. Bake uncovered for 12 minutes, or until the fish is opaque and flaky.

8. Serve warm.

## Turkey Bacon–Wrapped Halibut
(Serves 2)

>2 medium halibut fillets
>1 handful fresh rosemary sprigs, stems removed
>Juice and zest of 1 lemon
>Freshly ground black pepper to taste
>4 pieces of free-range, sugar-free turkey bacon
>Extra-virgin olive oil

1. Preheat the oven to 400°F.

2. Season the fish with the rosemary, lemon juice and zest, and pepper. Set aside.

3. Lay the bacon on a cutting board in two sets of two slices each.

4. Lay one fillet on each pair then wrap the fillets with the bacon. Cover as much of the fish as you like, or can.

5. On a large ovenproof pan, or on a baking sheet, drizzle a dash of olive oil, and set the fish in the pan. You won't flip them, so the side that's up is the side you'll serve up.

6. Bake the fish for 10 to 15 minutes, until it is cooked and the bacon is crispy.

7. Serve warm with another crack or two of freshly ground black pepper.

## Salmon Salad
(Serves 2 to 4)

2 6- to 8-ounce cans wild-caught salmon, or use leftover salmon from previously cooked fillets (leftovers that you have on hand)

2 celery stalks, diced

1 small red onion, minced

4 scallions, minced

6 tablespoons mayonnaise (make sure it's made with real eggs, not soy)

2 tablespoons miso

1 heaping tablespoon Dijon mustard

2 teaspoons chopped fresh dill

Sea salt and freshly ground black pepper to taste

1. In a medium bowl, mix all the ingredients together.

2. Serve in lettuce leaves, like a wrap, or on a bed of mixed greens for a delicious tuna-fish alternative.

## Fish and Chips
(Serves 2 to 6)

> 2 delicata squash, or 1 of any larger winter squash (acorn, butternut, kabocha)
> 2 tablespoons extra-virgin olive oil
> Sea salt and freshly ground black pepper to taste
> ½ cup almond meal
> ½ teaspoon chili powder
> 2 medium boneless cold-water white fish fillets, such as haddock or cod
> 1 egg white

1. Preheat the oven to 450°F.

2. Cut the squash into wedge-shaped fries. The skin is actually really delicious and nutritious, so we recommend leaving it on, but peel them if you prefer.

3. On a large baking sheet, toss the squash pieces with the olive oil, salt, and pepper until they are well coated, then spread them in an even layer.

4. Bake for 20 minutes, turn the fries over, and bake for an additional 15 to 20 minutes, or until they are tender and darkened. Remove from the oven.

5. While the fries are baking, prepare the fish. In a small bowl, combine the almond meal and chili powder.

6. In another small bowl, beat the egg white with a fork or whisk.

7. Dip the fish fillets first into the beaten egg white, then into the crumb mixture, then shake them gently to remove any excess, but make sure each is evenly coated.

8. Place the fillets on a clean, oiled baking sheet (not the one you used for the squash).

9. Bake for 10 to 15 minutes, until they are tender and golden but not overcooked.

10. Serve with the squash fries.

# POULTRY ENTRÉES

## Chicken Pot Pie
(Serves 4 to 6)

3 tablespoons coconut oil
3 to 4 shallots, minced
1 cup sliced carrots
2 celery stalks, chopped
6 garlic cloves, minced and divided into two equal
  portions
2 to 3 boneless chicken breasts (about 1½ pounds), diced
1 cup green peas, fresh or frozen
2 cups chicken broth (may need more but start with this
  amount)
Sea salt and freshly ground black pepper to taste
½ red onion, minced
1½ cup raw cashews, soaked for 4 to 6 hours, then drained
½ teaspoon cayenne
Optional: 1 teaspoon smoked paprika

*Crust*

1½ cups blanched almond flour
½ cup raw sunflower seeds
1 tablespoon dried herbs, such as sage, rosemary, thyme,
  or chives (fresh herbs will work too; just use a bit more)
1 teaspoon garlic powder
½ teaspoon sea salt
1 tablespoon extra-virgin olive oil
1 tablespoon water

1. Heat 2 tablespoons of the coconut oil in a large skillet set
   over medium-high heat.

2. Add the shallots and sauté them for 5 minutes, or until
   they are translucent.

3. Add the carrots, celery, and half the minced garlic, and continue to sauté until the carrots begin to soften, about 3 to 5 minutes.

4. Add the chicken and cook until most of the pink hue is gone from the flesh.

5. Add the peas and ½ cup of the chicken broth.

6. Continue simmering until the vegetables are tender and the chicken is fully cooked.

7. Salt and pepper to taste, and set aside.

8. In a medium skillet, heat the remaining tablespoon of coconut oil over medium-high heat.

9. Add the red onion and sauté 5 to 8 minutes.

10. Add the other half of the garlic and sauté for an additional 3 minutes. Remove from the heat.

11. In a blender, purée the onion mixture, cashews, 1½ cups of the chicken broth, cayenne, and the optional paprika until smooth.

12. Transfer the mixture back to the large skillet with the chicken and vegetables, and cook everything over medium heat until the mixture thickens, about 5 minutes.

13. Add more broth if needed and stir frequently.

14. Further salt and pepper to taste, then transfer everything to a lightly oiled deep baking dish.

15. Preheat the oven to 350°F.

16. To make the crust, in a food processor combine the flour, sunflower seeds, herbs, garlic powder, salt, olive oil, and water, and pulse everything until well combined.

17. Roll the dough out on a lightly floured (non-gluten flour) cutting board or on a sheet of parchment paper, which might be helpful in transferring the dough to the baking dish.

18. Lay the dough over the top of the chicken mixture.

19. Bake for 20 minutes or until golden brown.

## Turkey Chili
(Serves 4 to 6)

2 tablespoons coconut oil
1 pound ground turkey
1 yellow or red onion, diced
1 small winter squash, peeled and cubed
2 garlic cloves, minced
1 red bell pepper, diced
2 zucchini, diced
2 tablespoons chili powder (more if you like a little kick)
1½ tablespoons ground cumin
1 tablespoon paprika
1 teaspoon ground cinnamon
1 tablespoon raw cacao powder
1 24-ounce glass jar of tomatoes (Bionaturae, but canned
   is okay if this brand isn't available)
Sea salt and freshly ground black pepper to taste

1. In a stockpot set over medium-high heat, warm the
   coconut oil.

2. Add the turkey and sauté it until browned. Then add the
   onion and squash, sautéing until the squash is soft, about
   5 to 10 minutes. Stir frequently to prevent burning.

3. Add the garlic, red pepper, and zucchini.

4. Sauté an additional 3 minutes.

5. Add the chili powder, cumin, paprika, cinnamon, and
   cacao powder, and continue cooking until the spices are
   fragrant, about 2 minutes. Then add the tomatoes and
   simmer for an additional 10 to 15 minutes.

6. Serve warm.

## Almond Lime Chicken Stir-Fry
(Serves 2)

2 to 3 tablespoons extra-virgin olive oil or coconut oil
2-inch fresh ginger piece, peeled and minced
2 garlic cloves, minced
1 red onion, cut into thin half-rounds
2 medium carrots, peeled and thinly sliced on the
    diagonal
2 small boneless chicken breasts, diced or cut into thin strips
1 medium bunch Swiss chard (8 to 12 stalks), roughly
    chopped
2 tablespoons wheat-free tamari
Juice of 2 limes, or to taste
1 cup unsalted raw or dry-roasted almonds
Optional: sea salt and freshly ground black pepper to taste

1. Preheat a large skillet or wok over high heat. Once hot, add a few spoonfuls of olive or coconut oil and swirl it around.

2. Sauté the ginger, garlic, onion, and carrots in the skillet until everything is tender.

3. Stir in the chicken, cooking until it browns.

4. Add the chard, tamari, almonds, and lime juice to taste. Continue to stir constantly.

5. When everything is wilted, and the chicken browned, tender, and cooked through, it's ready to serve.

6. Garnish perhaps with chopped scallions or fresh cilantro leaves, and season with salt and pepper, if you like.

## Curried Duck
(Serves 2)

> 2 teaspoons sea salt
> 4 garlic cloves, minced
> 1 teaspoon cumin seeds
> 2 tablespoons curry powder
> 2 tablespoons extra-virgin olive oil
> 2 boneless duck breasts (substitute chicken breasts, if you prefer)

1. In a bowl, combine the salt, garlic, cumin seeds, curry powder, and olive oil.

2. Rub the duck breasts with the mixture until they are well coated.

3. Cover and let them marinate either overnight or for at least 1 hour in the fridge (the longer the better).

4. Preheat the oven to 450°F.

5. Place the duck in a lightly oiled baking dish and roast for 10 minutes, or until it's tender.

6. Serve perhaps on a bed of lightly steamed kale, chard, or some watercress.

## Sweet and Spicy Chicken Wings
(Serves 2)

> 3 garlic cloves, finely minced, or 2 teaspoons garlic powder
> Stevia to taste (probably just a tiny sprinkle will do)
> 2 teaspoons paprika
> 1 tablespoon wheat-free tamari
> 2 teaspoons unsweetened ketchup
> 4 small chicken wings (or thighs or legs, if you prefer)

1. In a baking dish, in which all the chicken pieces can lay flat, mix together the garlic, stevia, paprika, tamari, and ketchup.

2. Roll the chicken pieces around in the mixture until they are well coated. Then let them marinate for 20 minutes to 1 hour in the fridge.

3. Preheat the oven to 375°F.

4. Transfer chicken and marinade to baking dish. Bake the chicken for 45 minutes to 1 hour, turning once, until the chicken is tender.

5. Serve with the excess marinade, if you wish.

## Slow-Cooked Chicken Thighs
(Serves 2)

> 2 chicken thighs
> 1 teaspoon sea salt
> ½ teaspoon freshly ground black pepper
> 1 teaspoon ground fennel seed
> 2 tablespoons coconut oil
> 2 garlic cloves, minced
> 2 cups chicken broth (can also use homemade stock,
>     either beef or chicken; see recipes on pages 180, 191)
> 1 fennel bulb, quartered
> 1 cup chopped zucchini, cut into ½- to 1-inch cubes
> Sea salt
> 8 fresh basil leaves, minced

1. Allow the chicken thighs to come to room temperature.

2. Then season them with the salt, pepper, and ground fennel seed.

3. In a large skillet set over medium-high heat, melt the coconut oil.

4. Add the chicken, skin side down, and cook for 5 to 8 minutes, allowing the skin to become nice and brown.

5. When browned, turn the chicken and stir in the garlic. Cook until the mixture is fragrant, then add the chicken broth. Cover and simmer for 25 minutes.

6. Add the fennel and zucchini, cover again, and cook just until everything is tender.

7. Season with sea salt, and stir in the basil just before serving.

8. Spoon extra cooking juice and vegetables over each piece of chicken.

## Chicken Stock

1 whole free-range or chicken (organs, feet, gizzards, etc.
included if possible) or 2 to 3 pounds of bony chicken
parts, such as necks, backs, breastbones and wings
(important to use free-range, since factory farmed
chickens will not yield the same nutritious benefits)
4 quarts filtered water
2 tablespoons apple cider vinegar
1 large red or yellow onion, roughly chopped
2 carrots, unpeeled if organic, roughly chopped
3 celery stalks, roughly chopped
1 medium-size bunch of parsley
8 to 10 stalks rosemary (tied together with parsley)

1. If you are using a whole chicken, cut off the wings and
   neck and cut into several pieces for easier handling.

2. Place chicken or chicken pieces in a large pot with water,
   apple cider vinegar, and all vegetables except the herbs.
   Let stand for 1 hour.

3. Bring to a boil, and remove scum that rises to the top.

4. Reduce heat, cover, and simmer for 6 to 8 hours. The
   longer it simmers, the more flavorful it will be.

5. Add herb bunch when you have an hour left.

6. Remove whole chicken or pieces with a slotted spoon. If
   there is cooked meat on the bones, let it cool and then
   remove to use in other recipes (chicken salad, soups,
   curries, etc.).

7. Strain the stock into a large jar and keep in the refrigerator
   until the fat rises to the top. Skim it off and discard.

8. Keep stock in glass jars in the refrigerator or freeze in ice
   cube trays to store for later use.

## Garlic Lemon Chicken
(Serves 4)

> 1 lemon, quartered
> 5 to 6 sprigs fresh rosemary, bashed around a little with a
>    knife or in a mortar and pestle to release the flavor
> 4 tablespoons extra-virgin olive oil
> 2 garlic cloves, minced
> Pinch of sea salt
> Pinch of freshly ground black pepper
> 4 boneless, skinless chicken breasts
> 3 carrots, peeled and chopped
> 2 medium parsnips, peeled and cut into lengthwise strips
>    (the thinner they are, the faster they'll roast)

1. In a bowl, squeeze the juice from the lemon wedges and add the rosemary, olive oil, garlic, salt, and pepper, along with the squeezed lemon pieces. Set the marinade aside.

2. Slice the chicken breasts into about four pieces each, so you have sixteen pieces of chicken. Add them to the bowl of marinade and massage the pieces so each is well coated. You'll begin to see the meat curing in the lemon juice (turning white). It's best if it sits in the marinade for at least 1 hour, but several is even better. Store in the fridge.

3. Preheat the oven to 425°F.

4. Combine the carrots, parsnips, and the entire contents of the bowl of marinade along with the chicken pieces in a lightly oiled baking dish.

5. Cook for roughly 40 to 45 minutes, but keep checking, since oven temperatures and cooking times can vary. Just be sure the chicken is cooked through and the parsnips are tender.

6. Serve warm.

# LAMB AND BEEF ENTRÉES

## Lamb Chops with Rosemary and Steamed Asparagus
(Serves 4)

- ½ pound asparagus
- ½ teaspoon sea salt
- 1 tablespoon extra-virgin olive oil
- 1 small handful fresh rosemary leaves, minced
- 2 garlic cloves, minced
- 1 tablespoon Dijon mustard
- 4 lamb chops or 1 rack of lamb

1. Trim the woody ends off the asparagus. You may also peel off about 1 inch of the tough, green, fibrous sheath from the base of each asparagus stalk with a vegetable peeler, if you like.

2. In a saucepan, pour in a 3-inch depth of water and add the salt. Bring the water to a boil.

3. Blanch the asparagus in the water for about 3 minutes, or until tender but not soft—al dente. Drain the spears and set them aside.

4. Make a paste of the olive oil, rosemary, garlic, and Dijon mustard. Then brush each lamb chop with the paste.

5. Grill, sauté, or broil the lamb chops at a high heat for 3 to 4 minutes on each side until medium-rare. Then remove them from the heat.

6. Arrange the asparagus and lamb chops on a serving plate and serve.*

*For a delicious additional flavor note, roast some whole garlic cloves in a small, ovenproof dish at 350°F for 30 minutes and serve them with the lamb chops.

## Lamb Tacos
(Serves 4)

 2 tablespoons coconut oil
 4 ounces ground lamb
 1 medium summer (yellow) squash, diced
 ¼ cup minced red onion
 1 garlic clove, minced
 1 tablespoon taco or fajita seasoning
 Sea salt to taste
 Romaine lettuce (to use as taco shells)
 1 to 2 tablespoons chopped fresh cilantro leaves
 Premade guacamole
 Optional: fresh sprouts, for garnish, any kind

1. Heat a large sauté pan over high heat.

2. Melt the coconut oil in the pan and continue to heat the oil until it is lightly smoking.

3. Add the lamb and stir until browned.

4. After the lamb is browned, add the squash, onion, garlic, and taco seasoning. Stir well to combine all the ingredients and cook the mixture until the lamb is cooked through and the vegetables are soft.

5. Season with salt to taste.

6. Arrange a few lettuce leaves or tortillas on a serving plate.

7. Top with the lamb and vegetables, then sprinkle with the cilantro.

8. Add guacamole however you like and garnish with the optional sprouts.

## Zucchini Stuffed with Middle Eastern Lamb and Tahini Sauce
(Serves 2 to 4)

3 medium to large zucchini
1 tablespoon coconut oil
1 small red onion, finely chopped
2 garlic cloves, minced
½ cup pine nuts
¼ cup pitted Greek olives, chopped
1 teaspoon paprika (the dish is even better with smoked paprika)
1 tablespoon ground cumin
1 teaspoon ground cinnamon
1 pound ground lamb
Sea salt to taste
3 tablespoons extra-virgin olive oil

*Tahini Sauce*

2 garlic cloves
Juice of 2 small lemons
½ cup tahini
Optional: ¼ cup cashew butter (optional, but makes it a little sweeter)
Sea salt to taste

1. Preheat the oven to 375°F.

2. Cut each zucchini in half lengthwise and carefully scoop out the seeds and flesh, removing as much as possible while keeping the zucchini intact. Set aside.

3. In a large skillet set over medium-high heat, warm the coconut oil.

4. Sauté the onion and garlic until they are soft and starting to caramelize.

5. Add the pine nuts, olives, paprika, cumin, and cinnamon.

6. Sauté for an additional 2 minutes.

7. Add the lamb and continue to cook until the meat is browned.

8. Remove the skillet from the heat and salt to taste.

9. Use the olive oil to oil a baking sheet, and place the zucchini skin side down.

10. Fill the carved out zucchini boats with the lamb mixture.

11. Bake for 25 to 30 minutes.

12. While the zucchini are baking, make the tahini sauce.

13. Mince the garlic in a food processor, then add the lemon juice, tahini, and optional cashew butter, and process until smooth. For a thinner sauce, add small amounts of warm water until the desired consistency is achieved.

14. When the zucchini are ready, remove them from the oven, and serve them smothered in the tahini sauce.

# Shepherd's Pie
(Serves 4)

*Top Layer*
> 1 medium head cauliflower, chopped into florets
> 1 to 2 garlic cloves, minced
> 2 tablespoons coconut oil, melted
> ¼ cup plain almond, rice, or coconut milk
> Sea salt and freshly ground black pepper to taste
> Optional: chives or other fresh chopped herbs to taste

*Meat Filling*
> 3 tablespoons coconut oil
> 1 medium red or yellow onion, chopped
> 2 garlic cloves, minced
> 6 ounces baby bella or crimini mushrooms, sliced
> 1 large carrot, peeled and chopped (you can leave
>    unpeeled if organic)
> 1 celery stalk, roughly chopped
> 1 pound ground beef*
> 1 tablespoon coconut flour or almond flour/meal
> ¾ cup chicken, vegetable, or mushroom broth, or
>    homemade bone broth (see page 191)
> 1 tablespoon chopped fresh thyme, or 1 teaspoon dried
> 1 tablespoon chopped fresh rosemary, or 1 teaspoon dried
> 1 tablespoon fresh parsley leaves, minced
> 2 tablespoons wheat-free tamari
> Sea salt and freshly ground black pepper to taste

1. Preheat the oven to 400°F.

2. First, make the pie's top layer. Steam the cauliflower florets until they are tender.

3. In a blender or food processor, purée the cauliflower with the garlic and coconut oil, until the mixture is smooth.

4. Slowly add the milk until the mixture is still smooth but of a thick consistency.

5. Salt and pepper to taste, and add the optional herbs.

6. Set the mixture aside.

7. To make the meat filling, heat the coconut oil in a large skillet set over medium heat.

8. Add the onion and sauté until it's translucent. Then add the garlic, mushrooms, carrots, and celery.

9. Sauté until they start to soften.

10. Add the beef and sauté for an additional 5 to 10 minutes, or until the meat starts to brown.

11. Stir in the coconut or almond flour, broth, thyme, rosemary, and parsley.

12. Reduce the heat to low and simmer, stirring occasionally, for about 5 more minutes, until the liquid reduces and the sauce starts to thicken.

13. Stir in the tamari at the end.

14. Salt and pepper to taste.

15. Spoon the meat and vegetable mixture in a casserole dish.

16. Spread the mashed cauliflower in a layer over the top.

17. Bake for 35 minutes and serve warm.

*This can be made with lentils or lamb, depending on your preference.

## Hamburger Soup

(Serves 4 to 6)

2 tablespoons extra-virgin olive oil
1 large yellow onion, diced
2 garlic cloves, minced
1 delicata or acorn squash, peeled and diced
3 medium carrots, sliced into ½-inch-thick coin-size
   rounds
1 cup chopped mushrooms, any kind
4 cups beef or vegetable broth
1 pound ground beef
1 head bok choy, leaves and white stems chopped into
   large chunks
1 teaspoon curry powder
1 teaspoon paprika
¼ cup apple cider vinegar
1 tablespoon wheat-free tamari
Sea salt and freshly ground black pepper to taste

1. In a large soup pot set over medium heat, warm the olive oil.
2. Sauté the onion and garlic until they are fragrant and tender, then add the squash, carrots, and mushrooms, and 2 cups of the broth.
3. Sauté for an additional 10 to 15 minutes, stirring frequently, until the vegetables begin to soften.
4. Meanwhile, in a large cast-iron pan, brown the ground beef until it's tender, stirring frequently.
5. Then add the beef to the soup pot, along with the remaining broth, bok choy, curry powder, and paprika.
6. Raise the heat under the pot to high for 1 minute, then reduce it to low.
7. Add the vinegar and the tamari, and continue to simmer until all the vegetables are soft and beginning to fall apart, or at least cooked well.
8. Salt and pepper to taste and serve warm.

## Spiced Flank Steak
(Serves 2)

> 2 tablespoons apple cider vinegar
> 3 tablespoons chili powder
> 2 teaspoons ground cumin
> 1 tablespoon garlic powder
> ½ teaspoon red pepper flakes
> ½ teaspoon minced fresh ginger
> 1 large or 2 small flank steaks

1. In a small bowl, combine the vinegar, chili powder, cumin, garlic powder, red pepper flakes, and ginger.

2. Rub the mixture over both sides of the steak, coating it entirely.

3. Broil or grill the meat to your preference, rare, medium, or well done.

4. Serve as a steak or slice it into thin strips served over quickly sautéed dark greens, such as spinach, kale, Swiss chard, or bok choy.

## Grass-fed Stir Fry
(Serves 8)

> 2 tablespoons coconut oil
> 1 yellow onion, roughly chopped
> 1 garlic clove, minced
> 1 pound ground beef, grass-fed
> 2 teaspoons paprika
> 2 teaspoons minced fresh ginger
> 1 small bunch bok choy
> 2 tightly packed cups spinach
> 6 tablespoons wheat-free tamari
> Sea salt and freshly ground black pepper to taste

1. In a large cast iron or sauté pan, over high heat, melt the coconut oil. Reduce heat to medium and add the onion and garlic. Cook, stirring frequently until onions are tender and golden, roughly 4 to 8 minutes.

2. Add the ground beef, paprika, and ginger, stirring frequently to cook through.

3. After 6 to 8 minutes, add the greens to the pan, reduce heat to low and cover.

4. Let everything cook for 4 minutes and then remove cover, stir a few times until well mixed, and if the greens still need to be wilted, cover again for another 2 to 4 minutes.

5. Remove from heat when greens are bright green and wilted.

6. Season with salt and pepper.

7. Serve warm.

## Grass-fed Beef Bone Broth

One of the most digestively healing, nourishing and building foods available. It's good to make it frequently and always
have some on hand to consume as is or in recipes calling for
broth or stock.

> Approximately 4 pounds grass-fed beef marrow bones
>    (often labeled soup bones)
> Optional: 3 pounds rib or neck bones with meat
> Approximately 4 quarts filtered water
> ½ cup apple cider vinegar
> 3 yellow or red onions, roughly chopped
> 3 carrots, roughly chopped (unpeeled if organic)
> 3 celery stalks, roughly chopped
> 8 sprigs of fresh thyme and 1 bunch of parsley, tied
>    together with unbleached string (leftover tea bag string
>    works)
> 2 teaspoons black peppercorns, roughly crushed with the
>    side of a knife

1. Preheat oven to 350°F.

2. Place half the marrow bones in a large pot with the water
   and apple cider vinegar and let stand for one hour.

3. Place the other half of the marrow bones (along with
   optional rib and neck bones if using) in a large roasting
   pan and cook at 350°F in the oven until well browned and
   meat is tender. When done, remove from oven and add to
   the pot with all vegetables.

4. Pour the fat out of the roasting pan (save in a glass jar to
   use for cooking later) and add a cup or two of water to the
   pan, swirl to collect as much of the juice as possible and
   add this liquid to the pot. Bones and vegetables should
   be covered but with plenty of room (several inches) left at
   the top.

5. Bring to a boil. Check and remove scum that rises to the top. After skimming it off, reduce heat to low, add thyme and parsley bunch and peppercorns.

6. Simmer for at least 12 hours and up to 24. Remove bones with a slotted spoon and strain everything off so you are left with a clear broth.

7. Let cool in the refrigerator and remove the fat that rises to the top; you can discard or add to the rest of the saved fat for future cooking.

8. Transfer to smaller containers and keep some in the refrigerator for use within the week, storing extra in the freezer for later use. Freezing it in ice cube trays and storing the frozen cubes of broth in bags or plastic containers works well for reheating and easy serving sizes.

## VEGETARIAN DISHES

## Roasted Squash with Curried Tahini Dressing
(Serves 4 to 8)

   1 ambercup or kabocha squash, cut into wedges, with the
      peel left on
   Extra-virgin olive oil
   Sea salt and freshly ground black pepper to taste

*Curried Tahini Dressing*
   ¼ cup tahini
   Juice of 1 lemon
   Stevia to taste (be careful not to oversweeten)
   1 teaspoon curry powder
   1 teaspoon dill, fresh or dried (mince if fresh)
   1 teaspoon sea salt
   2 tablespoons almond or coconut milk (or water)

1. Preheat the oven to 450°F.

2. Place squash wedges on a baking sheet and drizzle them
   with olive oil and a dash of salt and pepper.

3. Bake until they are dark and tender (check with a fork),
   roughly 30 to 40 minutes.

4. Meanwhile, make the dressing. In a blender, purée the
   tahini, lemon juice, stevia, curry powder, dill, and sea salt
   until smooth.

5. Add enough almond or coconut milk (or water) to
   thin the mixture to your desired consistency. (Or whip
   everything together in a bowl until smooth, if you prefer.)

6. When the squash is ready, remove it from the oven and
   serve it warm. Either drizzle the dressing over the squash
   or serve the dressing alongside in small bowls for dipping.

## Pad Thai
(Serves 2 to 4)

1 small spaghetti squash
2 tablespoons coconut oil
1 red chili, chopped (use spice level to your preference)
2 garlic cloves, minced
1-inch fresh ginger piece, peeled and minced
1 large yellow onion, roughly chopped
1 small head broccoli, cut into florets
2 handfuls mung bean sprouts
½ cup chopped almonds
2 eggs
Juice of 1 lime, or 1 tablespoon lime juice
Splash of wheat-free tamari
Splash of fish sauce (Red Boat brand)
1 small handful fresh chopped cilantro

1. Scoop out the flesh of the spaghetti squash and place it in a bowl.

2. Heat a wok or large cast-iron pan over high heat.

3. Add the coconut oil, chili, garlic, ginger, and onion, tossing and sautéing until the onion becomes translucent and tender.

4. Add the broccoli and mung beans sprouts.

5. When the broccoli is bright and tender, possibly turning brown in areas, add the almonds and spaghetti squash flesh.

6. Add eggs, lime juice, tamari, fish sauce, and cilantro. Stir until eggs are cooked. Serve warm.

## Warm Zucchini Pesto Pasta

(Serves 2 to 4)

   2 tablespoons coconut oil
   ½ red onion, cut into ¼-inch-thick slices
   1 zucchini, peeled (leave unpeeled, if organic) and seeded,
      then sliced lengthwise into long strips
   2 heaping tablespoons dairy-free pesto
   2 to 3 tablespoons chopped olives, black or green or
      kalamata
   Zest of ½ lemon
   Sea salt to taste
   Freshly ground black pepper, roughly 4 to 8 turns of the
      peppermill, to taste

1. Melt the coconut oil in a large sauté pan set over medium-high heat.

2. Add the onion and sauté until it softens, 3 to 4 minutes.

3. Stir in the zucchini, then add the pesto and combine well.

4. Continue sautéing until all the ingredients are warm.

5. Stir in the olives and lemon zest.

6. Season with salt and pepper and serve.

## Thai Vegetable Salad Wraps with Almond Sauce
(Serves 4)

1 tablespoon almond butter
1 teaspoon grated fresh ginger
Juice of ½ lemon
1 teaspoon apple cider vinegar
1 garlic clove
1 teaspoon nama shoyu or wheat-free tamari
Pinch of cayenne
⅓ cup water
4 large Romaine lettuce leaves
½ head Napa cabbage, shredded
1 carrot, peeled and shredded
2 scallions, thinly sliced
6 snow peas, thinly sliced
1 cucumber, peeled, seeded, and thinly sliced
Fresh cilantro leaves, for garnish
1 package nori sheets cut into strips, ⅛ inch wide by 2
   inches long (The amount of sheets used will vary, so
   have a package ready; you won't use it all.)
Optional: thinly sliced almonds, for garnish

1. To make the almond sauce, in a blender purée the almond butter, ginger, lemon juice, vinegar, garlic, nama shoyu or tamari, cayenne, and water until the mixture is creamy. Add more water if the mixture seems too thick.

2. Set aside.

3. Wash the lettuce leaves and set them aside to drain.

4. In a medium bowl, combine the cabbage, carrot, scallions, peas, and cucumber.

5. Spoon about one quarter of the vegetable mixture into each lettuce leaf, roll up the leaves, and set the wraps on a serving platter.

6. Drizzle each wrap with 1 tablespoon of the almond sauce.

7. Garnish with cilantro leaves and strips of the nori or sliced almonds.

## Garlic and Summer Vegetable Kelp Noodles
(Serves 2 to 4)

8 to 16 ounces kelp noodles
2 tablespoons extra-virgin olive oil
4 garlic cloves, thinly sliced
1 large summer squash, cut into ¼-inch-thick rounds
2 handfuls mushrooms, any variety, sliced
1 fennel bulb, sliced
2 tablespoons chopped fresh basil, or any other fresh
    herbs you have on hand
Sea salt to taste
¼ cup pine nuts

1. Rinse the kelp noodles under cold water.

2. Drain and set aside.

3. Heat the olive oil in a large sauté pan set over medium-high heat.

4. Add the sliced garlic and sauté until it becomes slightly browned and fragrant.

5. Toss in the squash, mushrooms, and fennel. Continuously shake the pan or continue to stir with a wooden spoon to prevent the garlic from burning for 8 to 10 minutes.

6. Add the kelp noodles and stir for a few more minutes, using a pair of tongs to toss all the ingredients together.

7. Add the basil, letting it wilt, which should be just about when the noodles are perfectly warm.

8. Remove from heat and season to taste with sea salt.

9. Garnish with any additional fresh herbs and the pine nuts, and serve warm or cold.

## Garlicky Mashed-Up Frittata
(Serves 2 to 6)

> 2 parsnips, chopped into ¼-inch-thick coins
> 2 tablespoons extra-virgin olive oil
> 4 garlic cloves, minced
> 1 small bunch fresh scallions, chopped
> 4 tightly packed cups chopped kale
> 8 medium eggs
> ¼ cup almond or coconut milk
> 1 teaspoon sea salt
> Freshly ground black pepper to taste

1. Steam the parsnips until tender. Either peel them or leave the skin on, as you prefer. (There are tons of nutrients and fiber in the skin.) Set aside.

2. Preheat the oven to 350°F.

3. In a large cast-iron or other type of ovenproof pan, heat the olive oil over medium heat.

4. Sauté the garlic until golden and fragrant, stirring frequently.

5. Add the scallions and kale, continuing to stir, lowering the heat to medium-low.

6. Sauté the mixture until the kale is wilted and tender.

7. In a medium bowl, whisk together the eggs and the almond or coconut milk, then add the salt and a crack or two of black pepper.

8. Pour the egg mixture into the pan on the stove and stir to combine.

9. Add the parsnips and let everything cook, without stirring very much, for 8 to 10 minutes. Occasionally pull the vegetables and sides back so the uncooked egg mixture runs down to the bottom of the pan and cooks. But don't scramble the eggs. You want the whole thing to begin to set up.

10. Slide the pan into the oven and let it continue to cook for an additional 5 to 7 minutes. When the frittata is cooked through and the top is golden, remove it from the oven and either invert it onto a serving plate or let it cool in the pan for a minute and slice it into pieces.

11. Serve warm or cold.

It makes great leftovers for two to three days.

## Vegetable Lasagna with Cashew Cheese
(Serves 4 to 8)

*Noodles*

>4 medium summer squash or zucchini, sliced lengthwise into wide strips (roughly ¼ inches thick)*
>Sea salt and freshly ground black pepper to taste

*Vegetables*

>1 tablespoon coconut oil
>1 leek, the white part sliced into ¼-inch-thick rounds, the green part discarded
>2 portobello mushrooms, gills scooped out with a spoon, sliced into ½-inch-thick strips
>2 cups sliced crimini or white mushrooms
>1 medium zucchini, cut into ¼-inch-thick rounds
>2 garlic cloves, minced
>4 tightly packed cups of Swiss chard, roughly chopped
>Sea salt to taste

*Sauce*

>1 cup cashews, dry-roasted or raw
>Juice of 1 lemon
>1 heaping tablespoon miso
>1 teaspoon garlic powder
>1 to 2 teaspoons sea salt

1. Preheat the oven to 350°F.

2. In a medium bowl, toss the long squash slices with a fair amount of salt and pepper, enough to coat.

3. In a sauté pan, heat ¼ cup water.

4. Place the squash slices in the water, cover the pan, and gently blanch the squash until just tender, when you can lightly pierce each slice with a fork.

5. Remove the pan from heat and allow the squash to cool to room temperature, uncovered.

6. In another sauté pan, melt the coconut oil over medium-high heat, then add the leeks and sauté for 2 to 3 minutes before adding the mushrooms and zucchini.

7. Cook for an additional 3 to 4 minutes, then add the garlic and chard.

8. Using tongs, gently stir the mixture in the pan so the chard wilts without browning.

9. Season the mixture with salt and set aside.

10. To make the sauce, in a blender purée the cashews with the lemon juice, miso, garlic powder, and salt.

11. Slowly drizzle in up to ½ cup water as needed to create a smooth, creamy, cheese-like sauce. It's best to keep it on the thicker side so it stays put between the layers when baking.

12. In a medium-size baking pan (an 8 × 8-inch baking dish works well, or any pan you normally use to make traditional lasagna), create your layers. Spread a small amount of sauce in the bottom of the pan.

13. Add a layer of steamed squash slices, side by side.

14. Spread some cashew cheese sauce over those slices as evenly as you can and as thick as you like.

15. Sprinkle some of the vegetable mixture over the cheese layer.

16. Add another layer of cashew cheese.

17. Repeat the layers until all the ingredients are used up, topping with a layer of cashew cheese. There's really no wrong way to do it; some people layer the squash "noodles" first. It's up to you. Any way you do it will turn out delicious.

18. Bake 30 minutes, until the cashew cheese is browned on top and all the layers are soft and melted together.

19. Let the dish cool before you slice it into squares with a sharp knife. (A serrated steak knife often works best for this.)

20. Lift the squares onto serving plates with a spatula. Don't be alarmed if it falls apart a bit; it'll still taste incredible.

*To make the noodles, we like to slice the squash with a knife, since these need to be slightly thicker than if you were to use a vegetable peeler. If you do use a vegetable peeler or mandoline, be careful when moving the papery-thin noodles, since blanching makes them very delicate and they'll tear easily.

# SALADS

## Shaved Fennel Salad with Cheese and Herbs
**(Serves 2)**

¼ cup miso
¼ cup water
1 handful de-stemmed fresh dill (roughly 3 to 4
    tablespoons), or 2 tablespoons dried
2 tablespoons nutritional yeast
3 fennel bulbs, shaved or thinly sliced
¼ cup extra-virgin olive oil
Juice of 1 lemon
4 tightly packed cups mixed greens

1. In a bowl, mix together the miso, water, dill, and
   nutritional yeast to make a "cheese." Set aside.

2. In a large bowl, toss the fennel with the olive oil, lemon
   juice, and mixed greens.

3. When everything is coated, add the "cheese" mixture and
   toss lightly until everything is just coated and combined.

4. Serve with additional greens for a hearty salad.

## Acorn Wedges with Asian Kohlrabi Salad
(Serves 2 to 4)

　　1 large acorn squash
　　1 teaspoon extra-virgin olive oil, plus more for the squash
　　1 carrot, peeled and sliced into thin rounds or diagonal
　　　slices
　　1 small leek, the white part thinly sliced, the green part
　　　discarded
　　2 cups peeled and diced kohlrabi (can also use broccoli
　　　florets)
　　1 tablespoon sesame oil
　　1 teaspoon wheat-free tamari
　　1 teaspoon minced fresh ginger
　　1 teaspoon minced garlic
　　1 tablespoon apple cider vinegar
　　Sea salt and freshly ground black pepper to taste

1. Preheat the oven to 450°F.

2. Cut the squash into wedges, leaving it unpeeled, and
   place the wedges in a baking dish.

3. Drizzle the wedges with some olive oil, then place the
   dish in the oven, and roast the squash until it is just
   tender (when you can just pierce each piece with a fork)
   and turning dark, roughly 25 to 35 minutes. (I like the
   skin crispy but cook to your own taste.)

4. Steam the carrot, leek, and kohlrabi (or broccoli) until
   tender. Remove from the heat and uncover to stop the
   steaming.

5. In a small bowl, whisk together the 1 teaspoon olive oil,
   sesame oil, tamari, ginger, garlic, and vinegar.

6. Toss the steamed vegetables with the dressing.

7. Place a few spoonfuls of the vegetables on each serving
   plate, top them with the roasted acorn wedges, and season
   everything with salt and pepper to taste.

## Salmon Niçoise with Parsnips

A slight twist on the traditional, we use salmon and parsnips instead of tuna and potatoes.

(Serves 2)

   4 medium-size parsnips, peeled and roughly chopped
   3 tablespoons extra-virgin olive oil
   Sea salt and freshly ground black pepper to taste
   1 pint cherry tomatoes (if you can find sungolds, they're
      the best)
   Juice of 1 lemon
   8 tablespoons apple cider vinegar
   4 tightly packed cups arugula (roughly 2 cups per serving)
   2 6- to 8- ounce cans salmon, water or oil packed
   ¾ cup pitted kalamata or black olives

1. Preheat the oven to 450°F.

2. Arrange the chopped parsnips on a baking sheet.

3. Drizzle them with the olive oil, season with salt and pepper to taste, and toss them until they are well coated.

4. Roast them until they're tender, roughly 15 to 20 minutes.

5. Add the tomatoes to the baking sheet, toss with the parsnips, and continue to roast the mixture for an additional 8 or so minutes, until the tomatoes are tender and wrinkled.

6. In a medium bowl, whisk together the lemon juice, apple cider vinegar, and an additional splash of olive oil. (It's nice to use the olive oil left over when parsnips and tomatoes are taken off the baking sheet, as it's flavorful and warm.)

7. On a large serving plate, combine the arugula with the salmon and olives, top with the parsnips and tomatoes, and drizzle everything with the vinaigrette.

8. Serve immediately.

## Amazing Green Herb Salad with Black Olives and Dulse

(Serves 2)

> 2 handfuls baby greens mix
> 15 fresh cilantro leaves
> 15 fresh parsley leaves
> 3 fresh chive stems, roughly chopped
> 5 fresh basil leaves, torn by hand into smaller pieces
> 4 tablespoons roughly chopped dill
> 3-inch cucumber chunk, peeled and thinly sliced
> 1 red radish, thinly sliced
> ½ avocado, cut into cubes or sliced lengthwise
> ¼ cup sunflower sprouts
> 6 pitted black olives, sliced
> Dulse seaweed to taste (as a garnish)
> Extra-virgin olive oil to taste

1. Layer the ingredients, beginning with a base of the baby greens, then a mix of all the herbs (the cilantro, parsley, chives, basil, and dill), then the slices of cucumber, radish, and avocado, and top with the sprouts.

2. Sprinkle with the sliced olives and dulse, dress with extra-virgin olive oil to taste, and serve.

## Warm Wilted Kale with Chicken
(Serves 2)

  1 boneless chicken breast
  ½ to 1 teaspoon sea salt
  1 tablespoon coconut oil
  2 garlic cloves, minced
  1 large shallot, sliced into thin circles
  2 teaspoons capers
  2 to 4 tightly packed cups of kale, de-stemmed and
    roughly chopped (any variety)
  Juice of ½ lemon
  ¼ cup roughly chopped pitted olives (any kind; kalamata
    works well)
  Drizzle of extra-virgin olive oil

1. Cut the chicken breast into thin strips, and season lightly with sea salt. Set aside.

2. Melt the coconut oil in a sauté pan set over medium-high heat. Getting your pan nice and hot will help prevent the chicken from sticking to the pan.

3. Add the chicken strips and cook for 1 minute, then flip each one over.

4. Add the garlic, shallot, and capers, and toss gently.

5. Cook for an additional 1 to 2 minutes, then add the kale.

6. Pour the lemon juice over the kale, give a quick stir, and cover the pan.

7. Cook the mixture until the kale is wilted, about 2 to 3 minutes.

8. Toss in the olives, drizzle in a bit of olive oil, and add a pinch more of salt.

9. Serve warm.

## Baby Kale Caesar
(Serves 1 to 2)

⅓ cup raw or dry-roasted pumpkin seeds
3 to 4 tightly packed cups baby kale, or a mix of baby
    kale, chard, and spinach
2 hard-boiled eggs, peeled and chopped
3 to 4 tablespoons nutritional yeast
1 cup Butternut Squash Croutons
Clean Caesar Dressing (page 213)

*Butternut Squash Croutons*

1 small butternut squash, peeled, seeded, and diced into
    1-inch cubes
Extra-virgin olive oil, as needed to coat the squash
3 garlic cloves, minced
Sea salt and freshly ground black pepper to taste

1. Preheat the oven to 375°F.

2. For the croutons, toss the diced squash with the olive oil,
   garlic, salt, and pepper, then arrange them on a baking
   sheet and bake for 25 minutes, or until the pieces are soft
   and beginning to caramelize.

3. Remove the sheet from the oven and set aside.

4. Place the pumpkin seeds in a small skillet over medium-
   high heat (no oil is needed). Skip this step if using
   dry-roasted.

5. Roast the seeds until they start to brown and pop. Stir
   frequently and watch carefully to avoid burning them.
   Remove them from the skillet and set aside.

6. In a medium bowl, toss together the kale or greens, eggs,
   nutritional yeast, croutons, roasted pumpkin seeds, and
   dressing, and serve.

# Thai Chicken Salad
(Serves 2 to 4)

2 tablespoons coconut oil
1 shallot, minced
3 garlic cloves, minced
1 pound boneless chicken, cooked and then chopped
   or shredded
Juice of 2 limes
2 to 3 tablespoons fish sauce (Red Boat brand)
1-inch fresh ginger piece, peeled and grated
Stevia to taste
Optional: 1 to 2 teaspoons red pepper flakes
3 cups shredded Napa cabbage
½ cup grated carrots
½ cucumber, peeled and seeded, roughly chopped
2 scallions, chopped
12 fresh mint leaves, minced
¼ cup roughly chopped basil leaves
4 to 6 tablespoons fresh minced cilantro

1. In a medium skillet set over medium-high heat, warm the coconut oil.

2. Add the shallot and garlic, and sauté until they start to caramelize, about 5 minutes.

3. Add the chicken and sauté until the meat is fully browned. Set aside. Let cool, then chop or shred.

4. In a large bowl, whisk together the lime juice, fish sauce, ginger, stevia, and optional red pepper flakes.

5. Toss in the chicken mixture, cabbage, carrots, cucumber, scallions, mint, basil, and cilantro, and stir to combine. Serve immediately. This keeps in the fridge for 3 to 4 days.

# SALAD DRESSINGS AND SAUCES

## Walnut French Dressing

1 garlic clove, peeled and minced
1 heaping tablespoon Dijon mustard
2 tablespoons apple cider vinegar
8 tablespoons walnut oil
½ teaspoon sea salt
¼ teaspoon freshly ground black pepper (more to taste)

Puree all ingredients in a blender until smooth. Keeps for 3 to 4 days at room temperature in a glass jar.

## Curried Almond Sauce

¼ cup almond butter
2 teaspoons curry powder
1 tablespoon wheat-free tamari
Dash of sea salt, or to taste
3 tablespoons water

1. Blend the almond butter, curry powder, tamari, and salt together in a bowl or in a blender.

2. Then add the water slowly until the mixture is smooth and creamy. If you desire a thinner sauce consistency, add a bit more water, again slowly. This keeps in fridge for 1 week.

## Peppered Vinegar and Oil Dressing

¼ cup extra-virgin olive oil
¾ cup apple cider vinegar
1 teaspoon Dijon mustard
½ teaspoon chili powder
6 or more cracks of freshly ground black pepper
Pinch of sea salt

Shake all the ingredients together in a glass jar with a tightly fitting lid until everything is well combined. The dressing will keep for 1 week unrefrigerated.

## Sesame Dressing

2 tablespoons tahini
2 teaspoons chickpea miso
2 garlic cloves, finely minced
2 teaspoons sesame oil
1½ teaspoons lemon juice
1½ teaspoons onion powder
⅛ teaspoon mustard powder
⅛ teaspoon cayenne
Stevia to taste

Whisk all the ingredients together. Store in a jar in the refrigerator.

## Clean Ranch Dressing

1 cup raw cashews, soaked in water for 2 to 4 hours, then
drained (or dry-roasted cashews, also soaked)
3 garlic cloves, minced
1 teaspoon dried dill
½ teaspoon celery seed
Juice of 1 lemon
½ cup coconut milk
Sea salt and freshly ground black pepper to taste
2 tablespoons minced fresh chives
1 tablespoon minced fresh parsley

1. In a blender or food processor, blend the cashews, garlic, dill, celery seed, lemon juice, and coconut milk until the mixture is smooth and creamy.

2. Salt and pepper to taste.

3. Add the chives and parsley, and blend just enough to incorporate.

4. Store in a jar in the refrigerator.

## Clean Caesar Dressing

   1 cup raw cashews, soaked in water for 2 to 4 hours, then
      drained
   3 garlic cloves, minced
   3 to 8 roughly chopped anchovies (water or oil packed)
      to taste (start with 3 and add more if you like a stronger
      flavor)
   1 tablespoon chickpea or brown-rice miso
   1 tablespoon Dijon mustard
   ¼ cup nutritional yeast
   Juice of 1 lemon
   3 tablespoons wheat-free tamari
   3 tablespoons extra-virgin olive oil
   Sea salt and freshly ground black pepper to taste
   Water to thin, if necessary

  1. In a blender or food processor, blend all the ingredients
     until creamy, adding only enough water as needed for a
     smooth consistency.

  2. Store in a jar in the refrigerator.

## Zippy Lime and Cilantro Dressing

   Juice of 2 limes
   ¼ cup extra-virgin olive oil
   ¼ cup minced fresh cilantro
   1 garlic clove, minced
   1 teaspoon ground cumin
   Dash of cayenne, or more if you like more kick
   Stevia to taste
   Sea salt and freshly ground black pepper to taste

Whisk all the ingredients together. Keeps for 1 week in fridge.

# Resources

## Practitioners and Treatment Centers

Not all doctors are healers, and not all healers are doctors. Here are a few people who have helped Dr. Junger and the Clean team in their healing journey:

### Dr. Richard Ash
The Ash Center
www.ashcenter.com
Focusing on chronic illnesses, allergies, and joint pain, Dr. Ash is another Clean favorite. He practices in the New York City area.

### James Barry
(310) 876-2587
www.wholesome2go.com
Amazing Clean food delivered to your door in the Los Angeles area.

### Dr. Susan Blum
Blum Center for Health
www.blumcenterforhealth.com
A functional medicine and lifestyle education center in Rye Brook, New York, the Blum Center facilitates healing by combining treatment and skill building, helping patients establish healthy lifestyle habits for long-term success.

### Body Z Alive
1137 Second Street, Suite 205
Santa Monica, CA 90403
(310) 587-2639
www.bodyzalive.com
Great colonics in Santa Monica.

**Dr. Ilan Bohm**
635 Madison Avenue, 4th Floor
New York, NY 10022
(212) 277-4406
www.ilanbohm.com
Chiropractor, healer, and so much more

**Hugo Cory**
(212) 396-0020
Hugo teaches powerful tools to master yourself and clean your mind of quantum toxicity

**Nell Cotter, LMFT**
2730 Wilshire Boulevard, Suite 250
Santa Monica CA 90403
(310) 560–3240
http://therapists.psychologytoday.com/rms/name/Nell_Cotter_LMFT_Santa+Monica_California_83244
A marriage and family therapist in Santa Monica, California, with a specialty in couples counseling. Best I ever met.

**Dr. Gabriel Cousens**
Tree of Life Rejuvenation Center
www.treeoflife.nu
A place of healing and relaxation in Patagonia, Arizona, Tree of Life serves as a spiritual sanctuary, eco-retreat, lifestyle educational campus, and holistic medical spa. It specializes in type 2 diabetes treatments.

**Peter Evans**
(310) 721–6480
http://lifeprinthomeopathy.blogspot.com
lisa@peterevansinc.com
A gifted emotional healer, Peter Evans describes his work as taking the weeds out of your emotional garden. Incredible impact on people's lives.

**Gravity East Village**
www.gravityeastvillage.com
Gravity East is a center for healing that offers colon hydrother-apy, infrared sauna treatments, and nutritional consultations.

**Dr. Prudence Hall**
Hall Center Venice
hallcentervenice.com
Specializing in hormonal health from a functional medicine perspective, Dr. Hall is best known for her successful use of bio-identical hormones for treatment of both men and women.

**Dr. Bethany Hays**
True North Health Center
www.truenorthhealthcenter.org
True North offers integrative healthcare services in Falmouth, Maine.

**Dr. Mark Hyman**
Ultra Wellness Center
www.ultrawellnesscenter.com
An international leader in functional medicine, Dr. Hyman is dedicated to finding the root causes of chronic illnesses. In addition to writing several bestselling books, he works with patients at his clinic in Lenox, Massachusetts.

**Dr. Leslie Kaplan**
Pacific Urology Institute
2021 Santa Monica Boulevard, Suite 510E
Los Angeles, CA 90404
Great urologist. Kidney stone removal surgery.

**Davi Khalsa**
(310) 278-6333
www.tlcwomanscenter.com
Midwife, home births. Davi Khalsa has infinite wisdom in all areas of motherhood/pregnancy/birthing.

**Chris Kresser, L.Ac.**
chriskresser.com
A licensed acupuncturist and practitioner of integrative medicine, Chris is dedicated to spreading information about gut health and working with patients with chronic illnesses.

**Dr. Steven Levine**
2001 Santa Monica Boulevard, Suite 687W
Santa Monica, CA 90404
(310) 829-3350
Western medicine cardiologist with an open mind, great knowledge, and even better bedside manners.

**Dr. Amy Myers**
Austin UltraHealth
www.austinultraHealth.com
Dr. Myers has helped thousands of patients recover from chronic illness by changing their diet and healing their gut. She looks to find the root causes of illness rather than treating symptoms. Her functional medicine clinic, Austin UltraHealth, is located in Austin, Texas.

**Dr. Maggie Ney**
Akasha Center for Integrative Medicine
www.akashacenter.com
A naturopath specializing in women's health, Dr. Ney works with a team of holistic doctors at the Akasha Center in Santa Monica (Dr. Edison Demello and Dr. Myles Starr).

**Dr. James Novak**
Novak Medical Clinic
440 Lamont Street
San Diego, CA 92101
(858) 272-0022
Dr. Novak utilizes alternative healing therapies, like ozone and light therapies, to work with autoimmune diseases and other chronic conditions.

**Tracy Piper**
The Piper Center
www.thepipercenter.com
A standout colon hydrotherapist, Tracy Piper established a center in New York City to offer healing therapies, such as colonics, massage, acupuncture, and personalized nutrition and detox programs.

**Deborah Raoult**
(310) 625–3739
www.unfoldingbody.com
deborah@unfoldingbody.com
Doula, healer.

**Dr. Radi Shamsi**
Los Angeles Gastroenterology Clinic
(310) 453-0504
www.lagidoc.com
Western-trained gastroenterologist with an open mind. Also best for colonoscopies in Los Angeles.

**Dr. Rony Shimony**
Director, The Mount Sinai Heart and Vascular Midtown Center
485 Madison Ave, 17th Floor
New York, NY 10022
(212) 752–2700
Western medicine cardiologist with an open-golden heart. Dr. Junger's personal recommendation for anyone in need of a cardiologist.

**Sylvie**
Santa Monica, CA
(310) 458–3157
Psychic, medium, healer extraordinaire.

## We Care Spa

www.wecarespa.com

A dedicated detox retreat center in Desert Hot Springs, California, We Care focuses on liquid meals, elimination enhancement through colonics and massage, and lots of rest.

## William Wendling

(323) 356-3142

www.oxygenozone.com

Water filtration is very important. William Wendling not only has the best filters I ever found, but offers the best customer support on the planet. He can ship filters all over the world and work with your local plumber on the phone to assure proper installation.

## Women to Women

www.womentowomen.com

Dr. Christiane Northrup, a leader in functional medicine, cofounded this clinic in Yarmouth, Maine, and established a solid foundation in a holistic approach to women's health. She no longer practices.

• • •

You can visit the Institute for Functional Medicine to find a Functional MD in your area: www.functionalmedicine.org/practitioner.

# Recommended Reading and Films

**BOOKS**

*The Blood Sugar Solution: The UltraHealthy Program for Losing Weight, Preventing Disease, and Feeling Great Now!*
Dr. Mark Hyman
www.bloodsugarsolution.com
Just one of Dr. Hyman's *New York Times* bestsellers, this book reveals the importance of balanced insulin levels in preventing chronic illness such as diabetes, heart disease, and cancer. Dr. Hyman walks the reader through a six-week program addressing diet, exercise, supplementation, and more.

*Blue Zones: Lessons for Living Longer from the People Who've Lived the Longest*
Dan Buettner
www.bluezones.com
Explorer Dan Buettner traveled the world to discover why some cultures live longer, fuller lives than others. His book details the strategies for longevity found in these areas, known as blue zones.

*The Body Ecology Diet: Recovering Your Health and Rebuilding Your Immunity*
Donna Gates
bodyecology.com
A great resource for anyone attempting to heal the gut, with a focus on systemic fungal or candida infection.

*Breaking the Vicious Cycle: Intestinal Health Through Diet*
Elaine Gottschall
www.breakingtheviciouscycle.info
An introduction to the Specific Carbohydrate Diet, a therapeutic and restorative way of eating, which facilitates gut healing.

*Crazy Sexy Diet*
Kris Carr
kriscarr.com/products/crazy-sexy-diet

Kris Carr, cancer survivor and Wellness Warrior, shares her low-glycemic, vegetarian program, which emphasizes balancing the pH of the body with whole foods.

*Food Rules: An Eaters Manual*
Michael Pollan
michaelpollan.com/books/food-rules
Food guidelines made simple by one of the best-known food writers, Michael Pollan.

*Getting Real: Ten Truth Skills You Need to Live an Authentic Life*
Susan Campbell

*Hungry for Change*
James Colquhoun and Laurentine ten Bosch

*Loving What Is: How Four Questions Can Change Your Life*
Byron Katie

*A New Earth: Awakening to Your Life's Purpose*
Eckhart Tolle

*Nourishing Wisdom: A Mind–Body Approach to Nutrition and Well-Being*
Marc David
psychologyofeating.com
Marc David and his movement of the Psychology of Eating go well beyond a simple diet. In his book *Nourishing Wisdom,* Marc David explores our emotional and spiritual ties to food and gives the reader real steps to make lasting changes on an emotional and physical level.

*Real Food: What to Eat and Why*
Nina Planck
www.ninaplanck.com
Nina Planck makes food choices easy, championing traditional and whole foods, such as produce and good-quality meats and dairy, over factory-farmed and overprocessed "foods."

*Wheat Belly: Lose the Wheat, Lose the Weight, and Find Your Path Back to Health*
Dr. William Davis
www.wheatbellyblog.com
An in-depth look at how changes in food production and wheat farming coupled with our society's emphasis on "healthy whole grains" has actually fostered epidemic proportions of obesity and other health problems. Dr. Davis provides a sound argument for eliminating wheat and gluten from the diet for better health.

**MOVIES**

*Food, Inc.*
www.takepart.com/foodinc
A closer look into the food industry, uncovering what we eat and how it is produced.

*Food Matters*
www.foodmatters.tv
A collection of interviews with leading nutritionists, naturopaths, scientists, doctors, and medical journalists to expose scientifically verifiable solutions for overcoming illness naturally.

*Hungry for Change*
www.hungryforchange.tv
A look into the deceptive strategies used in the diet, weight-loss, and food industries.

*King Corn*
www.kingcorn.net
This documentary follows corn from crop to market, emphasizing the manipulation, overabundance, and gross overuse of corn, from corn syrup to animal feed, and how this is affecting the nation's health.

## WEBSITES

### Kris Carr
kriscarr.com
A crazy, sexy wellness revolution, Kris Carr's personal blog is a source of inspiration and great information.

### The Chalkboard
thechalkboardmag.com
A study in living well, this online magazine covers the gamut, from food to style.

### Clean Blog
blog.cleanprogram.com
A place for tips on Clean living and Clean recipes.

### Institute for Functional Medicine
www.functionalmedicine.org
A place to gather information, learn about upcoming trainings, or find a functional doctor in your area.

### Institute for the Psychology of Eating
psychologyofeating.com/blog/ipe-blog
Marc David's Institute for the Psychology of Eating addresses the emotional and spiritual aspects of food, with easy-to-use tips and tools.

### Mark's Daily Apple
www.marksdailyapple.com
A guide to the Paleo diet, with plenty of research to back it up.

### Mind Body Green
www.mindbodygreen.com
A wellness guide with countless contributing health professionals.

### Positively Positive
www.positivelypositive.com
An inspirational daily dose of goodness, with a focus on wellness and living a balanced lifestyle.

**Sarah Wilson**
www.sarahwilson.com.au
Easy-to-digest information on gut healing, nourishing diets, and recipes.

**Skin-Deep Cosmetics Database**
www.ewg.org/skindeep
This database offers practical solutions on how to avoid everyday exposure to chemicals found in cosmetics and toiletries.

• • •

Visit cleangut.com for many more resources, including a list of product recommendations, extra recipes, and shopping guides.

# Acknowledgments

*Thank you:*

To my wife Carla and my kids Grace, Judah and Uma Junger.

To my father, Alberto, who is watching and protecting me from above.

To my mom Muky and Herbert Donner. To my sisters Anabella and Andrea, and their partners Javier Rodriguez and Daniel Tugentman, and their kids Manuel and Clementina.

To the Clean team, Albert Bitton, Dhrumil Purohit, Kaya Purohit, Harshal Purohit, Hema Shah, John Rosania, Bonnie Gerlaugh, Robert Domingo, John Hand, Jessi Hinze, Jenny Nelson and Shannon Sinkin.

To my editor Gideon Weil.

A special thanks for Dhrumil Purohit and John Rosania for all their work helping me to write this book and for writing the guiding principles themselves.

And to all my patients and readers.

# Index

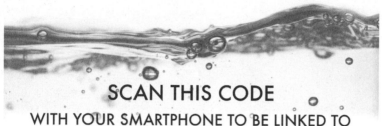

## SCAN THIS CODE

### WITH YOUR SMARTPHONE TO BE LINKED TO
### THE BONUS MATERIALS FOR

# CLEAN GUT

on the Elixir mobile website,
where you can also find information about other
healthy living books and related materials.

## YOU CAN ALSO TEXT

### CLEANGUT to READIT (732348)

to be sent a link to the Elixir mobile website.

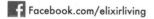 Facebook.com/elixirliving     Twitter.com/elixirliving     www.elixirliving.com